AEROBIC DANCE
A WAY TO FITNESS

Alternate Edition

Karen S. Mazzeo, M.Ed.
Judy Kisselle, M.Ed.
Bowling Green State University
Bowling Green, Ohio

Morton Publishing Company
295 West Hampden
Suite 104
Englewood, Colorado 80110

Copyright © 1984 by Morton Publishing Company

All rights reserved. The selections reprinted in this book are used by permission of and special arrangement with the proprietors of their respective copyrights. Permission in writing must be obtained from the publisher before any part of this work may be reproduced or transmitted in any form, or by any means, electronic or mechanical, including photocopying and recording or by any information storage or retrieval system.

Printed in the United States of America

ISBN: 0-89582-110-9

Edited by Dianne Kedro

Illustrations by Susan Strawn

Cover and photography by Clifton P. Boutelle and William Brown of Bowling Green State University News Service.

Acknowledgements

Special appreciation is given to the following individuals who have shared their time and fantastic talents to make this dream a reality: (Alphabetical Order):

BGSU and BG community students
Margaret E. Bobb
Clifton P. Boutelle
Richard Bowers, Ph.D.
William Brown
Steven Dunn, Ph.D.
Nancy Gilbert
Jane E. Herrmann (deceased)
Gwen Hyatt
Dianne Kedro
Tom, Kirt, and Keith Kisselle
Denise Marland
Dick, Mary Beth, and Michael Mazzeo
Lee Meserve, Ph.D.
Douglas Morton
Phillip O'Connor
Janet Parks, Ph.D.
Terry W. Parsons, Ph.D.
Virginia Retterer and "The Powder Puff"
Jane Steinberg
Susan Strawn
I. Clay Williams, Ph.D.

We wish to thank the following for giving permission to use copyrighted materials:

Kenneth Cooper, M.D., M.P.H., and M. Evans, Publisher
The National Dairy Council
Michael Newton, M.D.
Jack Wilmore, Ph.D.
United Feature Syndicate and Charles Schultz
Field Newspaper Syndicate and Erma Bombeck

CONTENTS

Preface v

1
Aerobic Dance: A Definition 1

2
Your Aerobic Dance Program 11

3
Posture: Where It All Begins 24

4
Warm-ups: Exercises and Routines 28

5
Performing Aerobic Dance Routines 45

6
Cool Downs: Exercises and Routine 47

7
Voluntary Conscious Relaxation 57

8
Choreographing Your Own Routines 64

9
Understanding Body Composition and Weight Control 68

10
Proper Diet to Complete Your Total Fitness Look 80

11
Special Populations, Concerns, and Misconceptions 90

Appendix: Evaluating Your Program 103

Notes 105

Index Card of Information: A Profile on You 109

Charts 111

Preface

Aerobic Dance: A Way to Fitness is an invitation to learn an exciting form of fitness through a sequential learning approach that uses a combination of exercise and dance called **Aerobic Dance.** This activity is gaining wide acceptance by all age levels from elementary school age children to senior adults.

Participating in a regular exercise program is an excellent investment of time. It may add to longevity of life, and it may significantly improve the quality of life. The final results of the aerobic dance program are a healthier, trimmer, more energetic you.

To date, there is no comprehensive text to fulfill the needs of the learner who is progressing through a course in Aerobic Dance, or a text for independent enthusiasts. To fill that void, this book has been developed by two educators who are specialists in the use of effective, creative teaching methods.

Aerobic Dance is divided into eleven chapters. The first two describe what aerobic dance is all about and give you the basic information needed for developing and executing a top-notch program. Chapter 3, detailing good postural technique, assists you with correct body alignment and efficient movement for the most effective use of the body during aerobic dance.

Chapters 4 through 7 dissect aerobic dance into the parts needed to make it a truly safe, challenging, and refreshing learning experience.

Chapter 8 presents the details for choreographing your own aerobic dances, allowing you **independence** to continue an individualized program.

Chapters 9 and 10 on Understanding Body Composition and Weight Control and Proper Nutritional Diet are included to give balance to the text. Lifetime assessment techniques and monitoring charts are also provided. To answer the many questions asked by individuals with special needs and concerns, Chapter 11 was created. And, completing the text, the Appendix presents a means of Evaluating Your Program. This provides various questions that you can ask yourself to assess the changes you have experienced over the past eight to ten weeks. The text concludes with reference notations and an Index Card of Information: A Profile on you, the student, to provide a means of statistical data gathering.

To our husbands, Tom Kisselle and Dick Mazzeo, and our children, Kirt and Keith Kisselle and Mary Beth and Michael Mazzeo, who proved to be quite "flexible" to provide the quality time needed to create this dream.

Also in loving memory of Jane E. Herrmann.

1
AEROBIC DANCE: A DEFINITION

"I'm gonna live forever!" is a line in a current, very popular tune. Some of us live our lives as if this were true — completely disregarding all personal self-discipline or pride in self and enjoying the easy life of overeating and underexercising. Our usual reasoning or excuse is lack of time. It usually takes a *crisis* situation to turn us around. But don't wait for a crisis! Set a priority — NOW — to develop a total fitness. Physical conditioning through aerobic dance won't guarantee you a longer life, but it *will* assure you a happier, more vivacious, and abundant one.

JUST WHAT IS AEROBIC DANCE?

Most simply stated, the term "aerobic" means promoting the supply and use of oxygen. The body's demand for oxygen will increase when you engage in vigorous activity that produces specific beneficial changes in the body. Aerobic dance is an exciting and challenging fitness activity that combines exercise (exertion) and dance steps (rhythmical movement). It can be totally individualized so that you can move rhythmically to whatever beat (rhythm), whatever tempo (speed), and whatever form of movement you enjoy most — be it jogging, jumping jacks, or jazz moves! The three main criteria for aerobic dance movement that you *must* include are the **duration** of time spent per session, the **frequency** of sessions per week, and the **intensity** (how stressful the activity is). The intensity of movement must be maintained at a certain heart rate (beats per minute) in order for it to be truly labeled "aerobic dance."

PRECAUTIONS

If you have refrained from regular physical activity for a long time, have recently had surgery, are thirty-five or more years of age, are obese, or have specific limitations, you need a physician's approval to start this cardiorespiratory fitness program, as you would at the onset of any new vigorous work or

AEROBIC DANCE: A DEFINITION

leisure activity. A thorough medical examination is the recommended way to make sure that your current state of health and your physical capacity are adequate to safely engage in an aerobic dance program.

AEROBIC CAPACITY IMPROVEMENT — YOUR MAIN OBJECTIVE

Aerobic dance significantly increases the oxygen supply to all body parts, including the heart and lungs, through continuous, rhythmic movement of large muscles and connective tissue. This type of movement conditions the body's oxygen transport system (the heart, lungs, blood, and blood vessels) to process the use of oxygen more efficiently. This efficiency in processing oxygen is called your "aerobic capacity" and is dependent on your ability to:

- Rapidly breathe large amounts of air
- Forcefully deliver large volumes of blood
- Effectively deliver oxygen to all parts of the body.

In short, your aerobic capacity depends upon efficient lungs, a powerful heart, and a good vascular system. Because it **reflects the conditions** of these vital organs, the **aerobic capacity** is the **best index (single measure) of overall physical fitness.**[1]

MEASURING AEROBIC CAPACITY

Pre-assessing your current status by having a thorough physical fitness exam will measure your heart's **response** to increasing amounts of exercise (work, stress) by measuring your ability to use oxygen.

Physical fitness can be measured in one of two ways:

- A laboratory physical fitness test
- A field test administered by you and a friend.

LABORATORY TESTING: SUB-MAXIMAL AND MAXIMAL TESTING

Sub-maximal testing is accomplished by means of a physical fitness test (also called a stress test) on a moving treadmill. Electrocardiogram leads transmit and record electrical (heart) impulses that are read on a machine and recorded on a strip of paper. You are tested only to 150 beats per minute — not to exhaustion.

The ECG leads are circular rubber discs that have wires attached to them. The discs are glued onto the chest and back at key locations so that various "pictures" of your heart — different angles and sides — can all be taken and recorded at once. Usually between three and twelve leads are applied, depending on the laboratory's procedures or on the individual's specific needs.

You will probably be asked to exercise (walk) at a pace of three miles per hour on the moving treadmill. The grade will begin flat and will slowly increase in gradation, as if you were walking up a hill. Every two minutes the "hill" will become steeper and more difficult to climb. When your heart rate reaches 150 beats per minute, a record is made of the **time** it took for you to arrive at that reading. Then, through an indirect method of extrapolation (projection of maximum results through having tested many others the same way in the past), your fitness ability is estimated.

Basically, the **longer** it takes your heart rate to reach 150 beats per minute, the more fit you are; the **shorter** it takes, the less fit you are. Sub-maximal fitness testing is usually used for persons who have no outstanding limitations known to them and who are interested in starting an aerobics program. **Maximal testing** procedures are administered if an individual's need is more specific (i.e., for diagnostic or research purposes). Maximum testing **directly** reveals how much oxygen you use, because you are tested to exhaustion.

FIELD TESTS OF FITNESS

You may not have immediate access to a laboratory and qualified physiologists to mon-

AEROBIC DANCE: A DEFINITION

itor the results recorded with the treadmill method. Therefore, included here are field tests that have been developed to help you assess your **own** physical fitness by determining your current aerobic capacity.

The following information and Tables I, II, and III were developed from Dr. Kenneth H. Cooper's book *The Aerobics Way*.[2] Cooper's Twelve-Minute Test and 1.5-Mile Test are two that you can administer by yourself or with the help of a friend. Assess your cardiorespiratory endurance using one of these tests before you begin your aerobic dance program. **Re-assess** your cardiorespiratory efficiency **eight weeks later.** As aerobic dance becomes a lifetime activity for you, plan an ongoing assessment every two months. Compare your results with those from your first assessment. This will also help you set continual, life-long specific physical fitness goals.

NOTE: If you are over age thirty-five, it is strongly recommended that you start an aerobic dance program by first seeing your doctor, and then having a monitored **laboratory**-fitness test.

FIELD TESTING GUIDELINES AND PROCEDURES

①

Before undertaking either of these tests, it is strongly recommended that previously physically inactive people participate in one to two weeks of walking and/or slow jogging before testing themselves.

②

Wear loose clothing in which you can freely sweat and a sport shoe that conforms to the guidelines suggested in Chapter 2.

③

Determine first **which** field test you plan to take — running with TIME **or** DISTANCE as the stopping point.

- If TIME is the stopping point, take the twelve-minute test.
- If DISTANCE is the stopping point, take the 1.5 mile test.
- If you feel rather strongly that you are really out of shape, the twelve-minute test seems to be easier because you run for only this amount of time. (It may take an individual twenty minutes to complete 1.5 miles.)

④

Be sure that you have a stopwatch or a second-hand on your watch, or that you are close to a wall-timer.

⑤

Immediately before performing the test, spend five to ten minutes warming up the muscles (see Chapter 4).

⑥

Run or walk (or combination) as quickly as you can for a total of **twelve minutes**/or **1.5 miles.** This is an "all-out" test of endurance.

⑦

When you stop, identify precisely the distance covered.

⑧

Be sure to cool off (Chapter 6) by walking slowly for several minutes and performing cool-down stretching.

⑨

Interpret results for the **specific test** and **location** that you plan to use (Table I, II, or III).

⑩

Record your data on the correct "Physical Fitness Appraisal" form (A, B, C, or D) and determine your fitness level.

Remember — for some beginners, the "good" performance level is very high. Do not be discouraged. You'll be pleased with your improvement as you participate in a **regular** aerobic dance program.

TABLE I
Cooper 12-Minute Run/Walk Test
Approximate distance in ¼ *laps* for a ⅛ *mile track* (190 yds.)[3]
Use Appraisal A

Fitness Category/Sex		Age 13-19	Age 20-29	Age 30-39
I. Very Poor	M	<12¼ Laps	<11½ Laps	<11 Laps
	F	< 9½ Laps	< 8¾ Laps	< 8½ Laps
II. Poor	M	12¼ - 12¾	11½ - 12¼	11 - 12¼
	F	9½ - 11	8¾ - 10½	8½ - 9¾
III. Fair	M	12¾ - 14½	12¼ - 13¾	12¼ - 13½
	F	11¼ - 12	10½ - 11½	9¾ - 11
IV. Good	M	14¾ - 16	13¾ - 15¼	13½ - 14½
	F	12¼ - 13¼	11½ - 12½	11¼ - 12
V. Excellent	M	16¼ - 17¼	15¼ - 16½	14½ - 15½
	F	13½ - 14	12½ - 13½	12¼ - 12¾
VI. Superior	M	>17¼	>16½	>15¾
	F	>14¼	>13½	>13

Key: < = less than
     > = greater than

From THE AEROBICS WAY by Kenneth Cooper, M.D., M.P.H. Copyright © 1977 by Kenneth Cooper. Reprinted by permission of the publisher, M. Evans and Company, Inc., New York, N.Y. 10017

TABLE II
Cooper 12-Minute Run/Walk Test
Approximate laps and distances for a .07 *mile track* (126 yds.)[4]
Interpreted from TABLE I. Use Appraisal B.

Laps	Distance	Condition of Women	Men	Both Age 30 and Under
10	.68	VERY POOR	VERY POOR	
11	.75	VERY POOR	VERY POOR	
12	.82	VERY POOR	VERY POOR	
13	.89	VERY POOR	VERY POOR	
14	.96	POOR	VERY POOR	
15	1.03	POOR	POOR	
16	1.10	POOR	POOR	
17	1.16	FAIR	POOR	
18	1.23	FAIR	POOR	
19	1.30	FAIR	FAIR	
20	1.37	GOOD	FAIR	
21	1.44	GOOD	FAIR	
22	1.51	GOOD	GOOD	
23	1.58	GOOD	GOOD	
24	1.64	GOOD	GOOD	
24½	1.67	EXCELLENT	GOOD	
25	1.71	EXCELLENT	GOOD	
25½	1.75	EXCELLENT	EXCELLENT	
26	1.78	EXCELLENT	EXCELLENT	
27	1.85	EXCELLENT	EXCELLENT	
28	1.92	EXCELLENT	EXCELLENT	

From THE AEROBICS WAY by Kenneth Cooper, M.D., M.P.H. Copyright © 1977 by Kenneth Cooper. Reprinted by permission of the publisher, M. Evans and Company, Inc., New York, N.Y. 10017

TABLE III
Cooper 1.5 Mile Run/Walk Test
Time (Minutes)
Use Appraisal C

Fitness Category	Sex	13-19	20-29	30-39
I. Very Poor	Men	**>15:31	>16:01	>16:31
	Women	>18:31	>19:01	>19:31
II. Poor	Men	12:11 - 15:30	14:01 - 16:00	14:44 - 16:30
	Women	18:30 - 16:55	19:00 - 18:31	19:30 - 19:01
III. Fair	Men	10:49 - 12:10	12:01 - 14:00	12:31 - 14:45
	Women	16:54 - 14:31	18:30 - 15:55	19:00 - 16:31
IV. Good	Men	9:41 - 10:48	10:46 - 12:00	11:01 - 12:30
	Women	14:30 - 12:30	15:54 - 13:31	16:30 - 14:31
V. Excellent	Men	8:37 - 9:40	9:45 - 10:45	10:00 - 11:00
	Women	12:29 - 11:50	13:30 - 12:30	14:30 - 13:00
VI. Superior	Men	< 8:37	< 9:45	<10:00
	Women	<11:50	<12:30	<13:00

Key: **> = more than
     < = less than

From THE AEROBICS WAY by Kenneth Cooper, M.D., M.P.H. Copyright © 1977 by Kenneth Cooper. Reprinted by permission of the publisher, M. Evans and Company, Inc., New York, N.Y. 10017.

UNDERSTANDING FITNESS TEST RESULTS

"Good" and "High" on the laboratory testing and "Good," "Excellent," and "Superior" categories on the field testing reflect that you are considered sufficiently physically fit to engage in a **continual** aerobics program.

If you place **below "good"** ("average," "fair," or "low") on **laboratory** tests and "fair," "poor," or "very poor" on **field** tests, you are considered physically unfit and in need of a **conditioning** aerobics program.

FITNESS FOR LIFE

Attaining a level of physical fitness entitled "good" or "high" (lab tests), or "good," "excellent," or "superior" (field tests) does NOT mean that you have achieved a finished product or goal. Instead, you have found a method of getting in shape that must be continued **for the rest of your life!** If you discontinue your program completely, all your aerobic gains will be lost in ten weeks.[5]

The need for personal fitness must, therefore, result in a complete change in life-style. You must prioritize and program exercise into your busy weekly schedule for the rest of your life. A "yo-yo" concept of a ten-week class now, and maybe one a year later, just doesn't maintain fitness and thus a healthy heart!

THE TOTAL PHYSICAL FITNESS PROGRAM

Total physical fitness is that positive state of well-being in which you have enough strength and energy to participate in a full active life-style of your own choice.

A **total** fitness program consists of three basic parts:

①

Aerobic (cardiovascular and respiratory) fitness (already explained)

②

Flexibility (ability to bend and stretch)

③

Muscular strength and muscular endurance training (thickening muscle fiber mass to enable individuals to endure a heavier work load)

More specifically, **flexibility** is the range of motion of a certain joint and its corresponding muscle groups. The greater the range of movement, the more the muscles, tendons, and ligaments can flex or bend. Muscles are arranged in pairs. One muscle's ability to shorten or contract is directly related to the opposing muscle's length or stretch. Flexibility is maintained or increased by movement patterns that slowly and progressively stretch the muscle beyond its relaxed length.

Muscular strength is the ability of a muscle to exert a force against a resistance. Strength activities increase the amount of force that muscles can exert or the amount of work that muscles can perform. Activities such as weight training can develop powerful muscles. Still, they do not provide a vigorous increased usage of **oxygen** to condition the **heart** to function more efficiently, as does aerobic activity.

Muscular endurance is the ability of muscles to work strenuously for progressively longer periods of time without fatigue. It is the capacity of a muscle to exert a force **repeatedly** or to **hold** a static (still) contraction over a period of time.

A total, well-rounded weekly fitness program should consist of regular participation in **all three components.** However, since the sign of genuine fitness is the condition of your heart, your blood vessels, and your lungs, **aerobic fitness** is the most important component.[6] By engaging in aerobic dancing (or any aerobic activity), your heart gradually strengthens and develops a greater capacity to pump more oxygenated blood to the body with fewer contractions (exercised hearts are stronger and slower).

Highly trained and conditioned endurance athletes have *resting* heart rates as low as 30-32 beats per minute, an unbelievably low rate! What actually happens is that with regular, stimulating exercise, the heart becomes a more efficient pump. It pumps more blood

AEROBIC DANCE: A DEFINITION

with each stroke, and with a more efficient stroke volume, your heart can function with less effort. By getting your heart into condition, you may be practicing preventive medicine. You may be lessening the danger of a coronary heart attack, five, ten, fifteen, twenty years from now. And if you do have one, your chances of surviving are far greater with a heart, and lungs, and blood vessels which are in good condition.[7]

It is thought-provoking to realize that you can still exist without big bulging muscles, or without the perfect figure, or with a head cold — but that you can't exist very long without a good heart and lungs. Unfortunately, more than 40 percent of all people who have their first heart attack do not receive a second chance to change their habits, or develop an aerobic program — they die.[8] And over one-half of all American deaths last year were due to heart-related diseases.[9] If only we could establish a living pattern priority **early** in life to correct this overwhelming statistic.

STRENGTHENING THE HEART: PROGRESSIVE OVERLOAD PRINCIPLE

Aerobic dance, like any aerobic activity, conditions the heart to **strengthen it** through a principle called "progressive overload." Not only will the heart pump more blood each beat, it will have longer rests between each beat, therefore lowering the pulse rate. Aerobic dance "overloads" the heart by causing it to beat faster during the vigorous workout, making a temporary high demand on the cardiorespiratory system. As you become more fit, the heart eventually adjusts to this demand and soon is able to do the same amount of work with less effort.

AEROBIC VERSUS ANAEROBIC DANCE

Very simply stated, all **aerobic** activity has several essential criteria that must be present in order for the exercise to be labeled "aerobic." Since "aerobic" means "with oxygen," the movement that you do must:

(1)

Use the **large** muscles of the body (like your arms and legs)

(2)

Be **rhythmic** ("one-two-one-two")

(3)

Be **continuous** for a twenty-to-thirty minute **duration** of time (actually, fifteen-to-sixty minutes, according to **intensity** — how stressful the activity is).

(4)

Be practiced for a **frequency minimum of three sessions per week**

- Four days a week or "every other day" is good.
- Six days a week is maximum. Give your body at least one day of rest.

(5)

And, in order to receive the cardiovascular fitness benefits, called the "training effect," the **heart rate must be maintained in a specific "training zone" or "steady state" — the individualized safe pace** at which to aerobically work or exercise. This reflects your **intensity** and is scientifically explained as a percentage of your maximum heart rate or maximum oxygen uptake. Intensity is discussed in more detail below.

Any activity that fits these five criteria above would be considered **aerobic**.

Anaerobic activity, then, is basically activity that is "stop and start," or one in which the heart is not kept at a constant steady pace for fifteen to sixty minutes or more. Thus, "anaerobic" describes an activity that requires an all-out effort of short duration and that does not utilize oxygen to produce energy. This type of exercise quickly uses up more oxygen than the body can take in while engaging in the exercise, causing an oxygen debt. This, in turn, causes lactic acids (waste products) to

8 AEROBIC DANCE: A DEFINITION

accumulate in the muscles, which leads to exhaustion.

WHAT IS INDIVIDUAL INTENSITY?

As briefly mentioned earlier, intensity means how stressful the activity is and is explained (or "measured" or monitored) as a percentage of your maximum heart rate. A specific individualized intensity is maintained by each participant during each session of aerobic dance. **The** intensity at which each individual works is **solely** determined by the individual's "steady-state pace," which is the estimated **safe** range in which to exercise. This is determined by your **age,** (unless you have heart problems or other specific limitations) and your **life-style.** Details for persons with limitations are given in Chapter 11.

TRAINING ZONE HEART RATE

This is the individualized safe area, or zone, in which to aerobically exercise — be it aerobic dance or any other aerobic activity. In order to receive the cardiorespiratory fitness benefits, called the "training effect," of any aerobic activity, the heart rate must be maintained in a specific training zone.

IT'S A PULSE MONITORED ACTIVITY

To insure that each individual learns how to **steady-pace** himself or herself for a **duration** (endurance) activity, learning how, when, and why to monitor the heart rate is one of the initial skills taught in aerobics programs. Once the pulse is taken, each individual records, on paper, what has been monitored.

HOW TO MONITOR YOUR HEART RATE

The pulse equals heartbeats per minute and can be felt and counted in one of six pulsation points. Select at which area you can best obtain a pulse, using your index and second fingers. The two places most often used for pulse counting are on the neck, near the carotid artery, and on the wrist, near the radial artery.

①

The carotid artery runs up the neck and is usually easy to find. Place your index and middle fingers below the point of your jawbone and slide downward an inch or so, pressing lightly. When you use the carotid artery pulse-monitoring method, make sure that you apply light pressure, as excessive pressure may cause the heart rate to slow down by reflex action.

②

The radial artery runs up the wrist on the **thumb side.** Place your index and middle

Taking the carotid pulse.

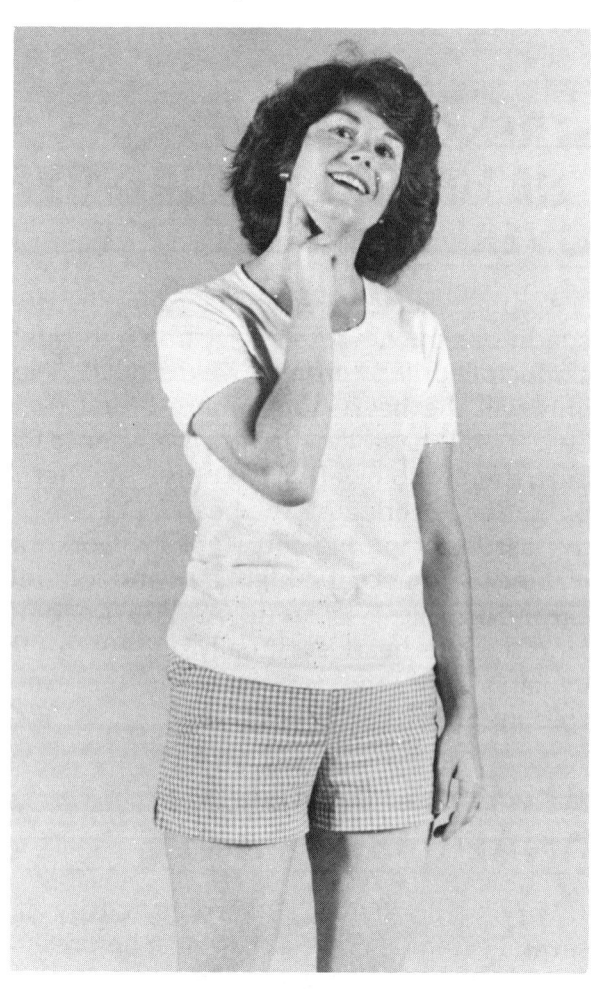

AEROBIC DANCE: A DEFINITION 9

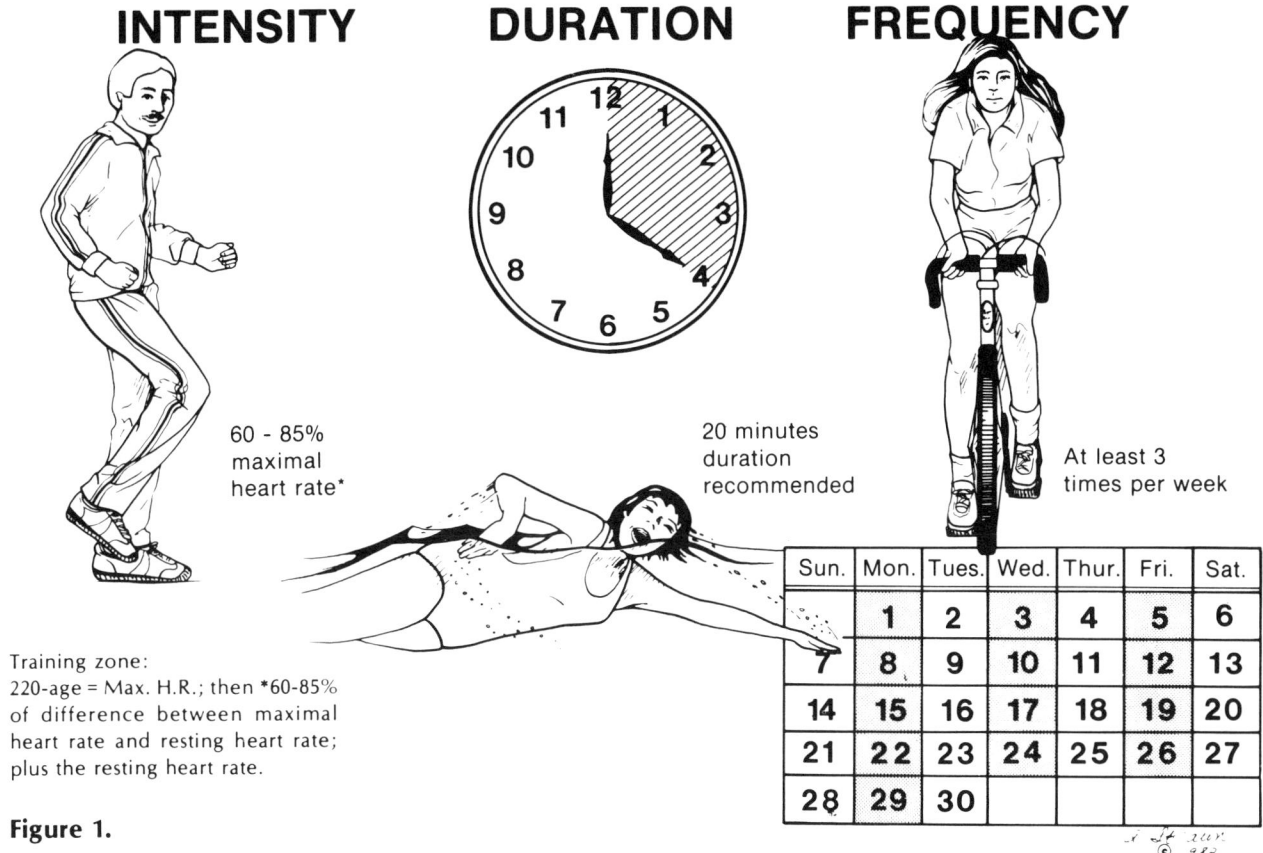

Figure 1.

fingers just below the base of your thumb. Press lightly.

Taking the radial pulse.

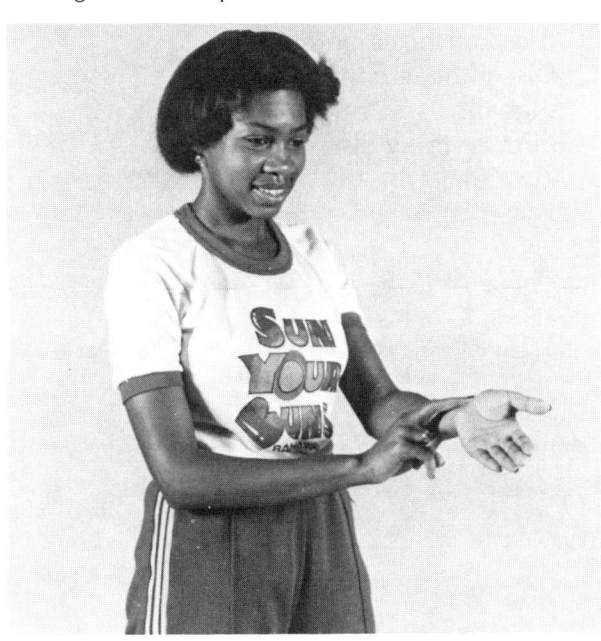

Now count the number of pulsations, or beats, for each six seconds and multiply by 10 (i.e., add a zero to pulse felt); ten seconds and multiply by 6; or fifteen seconds and multiply by 4. The total is the numbers of heartbeats per minute. To count correctly, make sure that you count each beat you feel.

Your heart rate will increase after vigorous aerobic activity and should return to normal within a short period of time after resting. As a rule, the faster it slows down (i.e., recovers from exercise), the more physically fit you are!

YOUR GOAL: TO ACHIEVE THE TRAINING EFFECT

By "overloading" the heart with vigorous aerobic dancing, your aerobic capacity is increased and a desirable **training effect** can be achieved. The training effect, or total beneficial changes that usually occur are:

- Stronger heart sending more oxygenated blood to all tissues of the body
- More blood cells produced
- Slower resting heart rate
- Expansion of blood vessels
- Improvement of muscle tone
- A lowering of blood pressure for some through improved circulation
- Stronger respiratory muscles
- Regulates the release of adrenalin
- Increased lung capacity
- A more regular elimination of solid wastes
- Lower levels of fat found in blood[10]

Other aerobic activities with which you can supplement your **aerobic dance** program include:
- Bench stepping
- Cross-country skiing
- Cycling (includes stationary cycling)
- Jogging/Running
- Jumping Rope
- Rowing
- Swimming
- Walking (moderate to fast pace)

Like aerobic dance, these vigorous, continuous, and rhythmic activities are excellent because they condition the cardiorespiratory system and increase its efficiency by demanding large amounts of oxygen over an extended period of time. The more you participate in aerobic dancing or other aerobic activities, the better your heart adapts to stress (by regulating the release of adrenalin) and works with the lungs to pump more oxygen to the muscles and body tissues quickly. This explains why cardiorespiratory (heart, lungs, vessels) efficiency is the most important component of physical fitness.

BENEFITS OF AEROBIC DANCE

Achieving the training effect, and therefore numerous beneficial physiological changes, will carry over into all of your daily living. A high fitness level will give you more energy to live life to its fullest. Once on the path toward fitness, you will be able to handle stressful situations, daily tasks, and emergencies better than before. Your mental capabilities — including better concentration —will also improve. You will have established a self-discipline toward keeping unwanted fat pounds away — that is, if your eating habits have been improved! And, as you incorporate correct posture through correct (efficient) aerobic dance movement, you will be working toward eliminating sagging abdominal muscles and toward strengthening weak back muscles associated with lower back pain. This new efficiency will then, very naturally, carry over into **all** of your daily work and leisure activities, providing you with a more comfortable, quality day.

People who engage in a **regular** program of aerobic dance will tell you from their own experience that they look and feel much better about themselves! As you begin achieving your fitness goals, the feeling of pride in yourself will surface and do wonders to boost your self-confidence. And, as you feel more positive about **yourself,** you will also develop a more positive attitude **toward others.** Just think what a fantastic impact this one particular fitness benefit can have on your life!

All of the above are incentives for starting and continuing aerobic dance. As you can see, the benefits are quite numerous!

There is nothing more difficult
than working against the flesh . . .
If you are successful,
it establishes a permanent
Discipline, a confidence,
that allows you to do well
in **everything** else you try.

2

YOUR AEROBIC DANCE PROGRAM

No wonder there is such a growing interest in **aerobic** dance. You have fun while you gain physiological AND psychological benefits. You achieve a good feeling about yourself and develop a more positive self-image. Students of aerobic dance have so much fun that they sometimes forget they are actually exercising and participating in one of the most effective physical fitness programs available today. Also, aerobic dancing has the necessary elements to prevent exercise from becoming boring and tedious.

Remember — the main objective of an aerobic dance program is to increase the maximum amount of oxygen that the body can process within a given time, thus improving cardiorespiratory fitness. Your body's aerobic capacity is dependent upon your ability to:

- Rapidly breathe large amounts of air
- Forcefully deliver large volumes of blood
- Effectively deliver oxygen to all parts of the body.

In other words, your aerobic capacity is dependent upon efficient lungs, heart, and blood vessels. Aerobic dance helps to develop this efficient oxygen transport system.

THE FOUR-SEGMENT AEROBIC DANCE PROGRAM

There are four essential aspects of a good aerobic dance program:

- A warm-up
- Aerobic dance routines
- A cool-down
- Relaxation

Warm-Up

Execute the warm-up stretching exercises with efficient posture for at least five, preferably ten minutes, in the order in which they are presented. As you warm up, you make all parts of your body more supple (Chapter 4).

②

Aerobic Dance Routines

Again using efficient posture, start with one routine and learn a new one **after** you have mastered the first one. Learn at your own pace. As you confidently execute one dance without hesitation or stopping, begin learning the next dance. Learning in the order in which they appear in the book is recommended. Once you have mastered these dances, it's time to develop your own (Chapter 8). Keep dancing and keep moving in order to reach your training zone and therefore work toward experiencing and obtaining the training effect. "Overload" your heart so that cardiorespiratory fitness becomes a reality. Start with several minutes and keep adding as much time as you comfortably can until you've engaged in twenty minutes of aerobic dancing. Working constantly in (approximately) three minute **intervals,** with heart rate monitoring in between, will allow the new **unconditioned** dancer a safe way to begin exercising.

If aerobic dance is new to you, **but** you begin at a **high** level of fitness (pretest out to be in "good" or better condition on a fitness test), your program can be of a **continual** high-intensity nature. Perform a minimum amount of heart rate monitoring. If you are in a conditioning course where the group works in intervals and/or frequently monitors the dancing heart rate, **you** engage instead in a high-intensity activity like jogging, jumping rope, reviewing what you've learned, or improvising movement that you enjoy (see Chapter 8 for ideas).

③

Cool Down

Choose an activity and stretching exercises that slow down large muscle activity (Chapter 6). Begin by walking for a minute or two, followed by **sitting** and then **lying** down while performing stretching exercises. If you complete a session by learning a new routine in which you are just "walking" through it, you can count this activity as part of your cool-down. A **minimum** of **five minutes** is required for cool down. Heart rate should be below 120 when you finish.

④

Relaxation

The Voluntary Conscious Relaxation Technique given in Chapter 7 totally uses your powers of control through your **imagination** — your **mind** seeks out and recognizes tension in a four-phase process. This brings a refreshing conclusion to a physically challenging aerobic dance session. Be sure to give yourself these five or ten minutes (or more) to complete the whole energizing process of an aerobic hour.

REMEMBER TO MAKE IT CONTINUALLY AEROBIC

You will find as you progress with your program that you will increase:

①

The **duration** — lengthening the time of each aerobic segment of your workout; i.e., from twenty to forty minutes

②

The **frequency** — from the minimum of three days to a maximum of six days per week

③

The **intensity** — gradually moving from the lower end of your training zone up to the top of your training zone by rhythmically and continuously using your large muscle groups in an increasingly more tense and firm fashion.

REMEMBER: Dancing at a high level of exertion for at least twenty minutes on a regular basis of at least three times a week is the key to an optimal level of fitness!

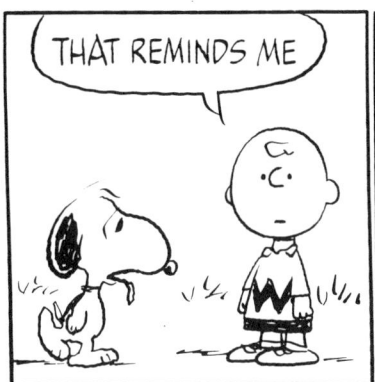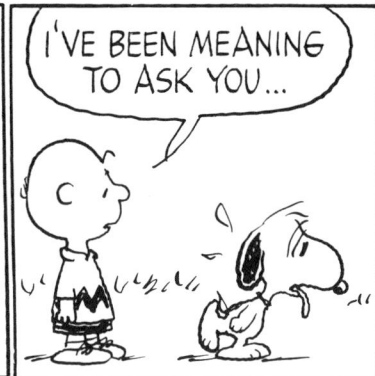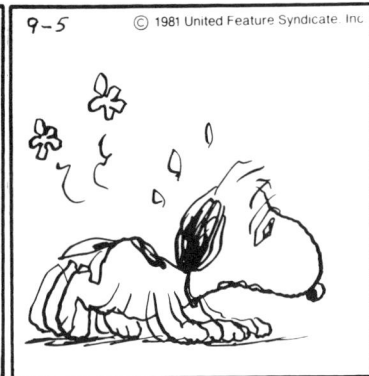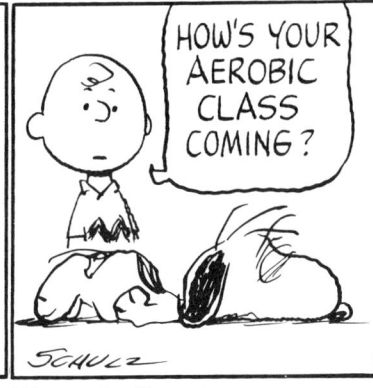

© 1981 United Feature Syndicate, Inc.

GRADUAL, SENSIBLE — DON'T OVERLOAD

It takes a planned self-discipline to become and stay physically fit, but the dividends of wellness and vitality are well worth it.

Progress gradually and sensibly in your sessions. Remember to warm up and cool down and to progress from easy to hard — both in the stretches and the dances. Learn to read your body signs. You're going to perspire and you're going to tire **a little,** but keep pushing. However, you needn't push to the point of discomfort. Know that an effective aerobic dance program may have some initial slight discomfort, so be sensible about pacing yourself. For example, after an aerobic dance, you may be short of breath, but this should subside within minutes after the activity. If it doesn't subside, you've worked too hard. If you are unsure about a particular discomfort or pain, ask a reliable person (such as your doctor) before you continue with the activity.

DEFINITE SIGNS OF OVEREXERTION

Remember — while monitoring your pulse helps you determine how hard to exercise your body, you also need to be aware of your own bodily signs. Signs of overexertion are:

- Severe breathlessness
- Poor heart rate response (monitoring too high a dancing heart rate, or final recovery rate not below 120 beats per minute after five minutes of cool down)
- Undue fatigue during exercise and inability to recover from a workout later in the day
- Inability to sleep at night
- Persistent severe muscle soreness. (The type of muscle soreness to guard against is not the immediate type, but that which becomes apparent after twenty-four to forty-eight hours.[1] Refer to Chapter 11 for details.
- Nausea, feeling faint, dizziness
- Tightness or pains in the chest

These symptoms do not mean that you should not exercise; rather, they suggest performing a reduced level of activity until you develop the capacity to handle more intense workouts. It is important to embark on an exercise program cautiously and to increase gradually the duration, frequency, and/or intensity of the program.

If you have any of these symptoms, ease down to a slow walk, sit down with your head between your knees, or lie down on your back and elevate your feet. This will help the blood move to your head more easily and carry the needed oxygen to your brain. If any of these symptoms last longer than a brief period of time, contact your doctor.

NOTE: Seek medical advice immediately and before the next exercise session if any of these symptoms occur:

①

Abnormal heart action

- Pulse becoming irregular
- Fluttering, jumping, or palpitations in chest or throat
- Sudden burst of rapid heartbeats

- Sudden, very slow pulse when a moment before it had been on target (immediate or delayed)

②

Pain or pressure in the center of the chest or the arm or throat precipitated by exercise or following exercise (immediate or delayed)

③

Dizziness, light-headedness, sudden incoordination, confusion, cold sweat, glassy stare, pallor, blueness, or fainting (immediate).

Do not try to cool down. Stop exercise and lie down with your feet elevated, or put your head down between your legs until the symptoms pass.[2] Information for various problems that frequent this activity are discussed in Chapter 11, under "Special Concerns, Care, and Prevention of Injuries."

SELF DISCIPLINE: A CHOICE

It takes hard work to achieve physical fitness. There are no shortcuts or easy ways. Once achieved, you must keep working to maintain fitness for life. **Maintaining** fitness is a lot easier than initially **achieving** it. The less physically fit you are, the longer it will take to achieve fitness. You will need to count your progress in months as well as days. Fitness requires self-discipline and choices. **You** are in control — no one or nothing else can do it for you.

THE KEY: ENJOYMENT AND REGULARITY

The key to maintaining a fitness program is to choose an aerobic activity that you truly enjoy and in which you can participate with enthusiasm and on a regular basis **for a lifetime. Consistency** is the **key** word. Remember that you can combine aerobic activities. For example, you can take an aerobic dance course that meets twice a week, then go for a brisk walk for your third activity. Or for your third activity you could run in place five minutes, jump rope for three minutes, and dance aerobically (that means lots of bouncing) for twelve minutes to reach your twenty-minute minimum aerobic program.

Now and then, exercise — no matter how enthusiastically engaged in — will not build or maintain fitness. We all have days when we don't feel like exercising. That's normal. Choosing an activity that you like most of the time will help you make exercising on the "down" days less of a chore. We think that's why you have chosen aerobic dance!

As you prepare your program, establish the following guidelines to insure yourself success:

①

Assess fitness in the beginning

Discuss your plans with your doctor. Sudden exertion could be enough of a shock to your cardiorespiratory system to lead to serious complications. Have a physical examination that gives you a complete understanding of your current health status and that provides guidelines or limitations. (See Chapter 11 under "Special Populations" for specific questions to ask.) Determine fitness level by means of a stress test (fitness test).

②

Set realistic goals

Make sure that they are goals you can reach. Write a self-contract covering one month for starters. Agree with yourself that you will set aside one hour, three times a week for your aerobic dance program. For many, a beginning level of fitness can be obtained in 8-10 weeks, if all aerobic criteria are used. Give yourself the gift of patience, for fitness will take *time*. It's all worth it though and the dividends are many!

③

Plan time on a weekly basis

There is no undesirable time other than immediately **after** eating. Early morning before breakfast and shower can be a good time. It is too easy to make excuses later in the day as you become caught up in the daily routine of responsibilities. Also, strenuous exercising just before eating will help decrease your appetite. If, however, you like to use aerobic dance to release the stresses of the day, noon time or before the evening meal are other opportune times.

Develop your skill at pulse taking

At the beginning of an aerobic program, learn to take resting, exercising, recovery, and relaxation pulses accurately using one of the six pulsation points. Resting, recovery, and relaxation pulses are most accurate by timing the pulse for at least fifteen seconds (and multiplying by four or more. Pulse taking during aerobic exercise is most accurate by an immediate count for six or ten seconds (and multiplying by ten or six, respectively).

Chart your progress

By monitoring on paper all aspects of your program, you provide a progress report with immediate feedback for yourself. Monitor and chart progress on the following:

- Resting heart rate
- Heart rates during your program
- Your weight maintenance, loss, or gain (details and procedures in Chapter 9)
- Your dietary intake (details and procedures in Chapter 10).

You also may enjoy keeping a running log or journal on your mental and emotional changes. After you complete eight to ten weeks of dancing, list all of your results (see Appendix). This will provide a "bird's-eye view" of your total progress to date!

MONITORING THE RESTING PULSE RATE

One of the two visible signs of **improvement** in heart and lung fitness that you can see happen on paper is a **lowering** of the resting heart rate. A true "resting" heart rate (RsHR) is not taken in a class but when the individual has been at complete rest (i.e., sleeping) for several hours and just awakens. Keep a clock or watch with a second hand next to your bed. When you awaken (without an alarm clock ring), take your pulse for a **full minute** and record that number as your RsHR (or for thirty seconds and multiply by two; or for fifteen seconds and multiply by four). Do this for **five consecutive mornings,** then determine an average (add all RsHR's and divide by five). This is a rather accurate determination of your resting heart rate.

NOTE: Unusual stress and **illness** (illness is a type of stress) will sharply **raise** the resting heart rate from previous readings. You will understand why it is so important, then, for normally healthy individuals to find a **positive outlet** for stress, for it affects you even as you sleep (constant rapid heart rate).

Use Chart III for recording your resting heart rate. The first week, take five (5) consecutive daily readings, and record this as your initial RsHR. Record your RsHR twice a week thereafter until the conclusion of the eight-to-ten-week course. Record your final reading below your initial reading and determine the loss or gain in RsHR for the eight-to-ten-week period.

MONITORING AND CHARTING DURING VARIOUS SEGMENTS OF AN AEROBIC DANCE SESSION

Two procedures are detailed here. Choose which best fits your needs.

See perforated charts at the end of the book.

USING CHART IV A

In the first column, register the date. In the second column, record your pulse rate before you start your warm-up and aerobic activity.

In the third column, record the activity and define it (i.e., **3 min. walk,** jog, or Celebration dance, 2:09 min.). In the fourth column, record the pulse reading taken immediately after the activity described in column three.

It is important to learn to pace yourself during your aerobic dance session. You are the only one who can tell if you are working hard enough or if you are overworking as determined by your pulse readings and your body signs. For example, if you haven't reached your steady state but feel fatigued, slow your pace down by "walking" through the dance or by actually walking about the exercise area, not even trying to move to the tempo set by the music.

Finally, in the fifth column, record your pulse reading taken after the cool-down and relaxation segments of your program. This pulse reading needs to be 120 or lower for sufficient pulse rate recovery after strenuous aerobic exercise. If your recovery pulse reading is over 120, it is a sign that you have overexerted yourself during this aerobic dance session. Therefore, continue with cool-down and relaxation exercises and your easy breathing pattern until your recovery rate **is** below 120. This **recovery** heart (pulse) rate is a second indicator of your physical fitness level (along with resting heart rate).

See perforated charts at the end of the book.

USING CHART IV B

Initially (usually for the first two weeks), readings are taken **after every type of exertion** (exercise) so that the individual develops an accurate skill of reading the pulse.

①

Pre-Activity Pulse Rate

According to what you've just been doing prior to class, this reading will greatly vary from day to day and from individual to individual. Take this reading on your **own,** for six seconds, add a zero, and record. It will give you a starting point for this session.

②

After (Independent) Flexibility Exercises

This is only done the initial two weeks to demonstrate that independent stretching is **NOT aerobic** activity, but escalates your heart rate slowly toward the full working range.

③

After the Warm-up Dance

The warmup dance will demand a stretching pace or tempo now higher than the independent stretching. The pulse will read a bit higher and will demonstrate that a **stretching routine** to music is also **NOT aerobic** — the heart rate will not be in the training zone. If you are really out of shape or have limitations, it will clearly demonstrate to you that your "aerobic" dancing will have to be at the lower end of your training zone in order for you to keep up for a twenty-minute (+) duration. Take your pulse for six seconds, add a zero, and record.

④

After the Warm-up Jog or Jumping Rope

This activity and pulse reading are included to fully get your heart rate up to the training zone, or a "steady-state pace." Your jog/rope jumping pace must be one in which you can endure for three-to-five minutes of background music, or of a song being played. If you can carry on a conversation with someone or sing the tune, it is the right pace. Don't run all-out and then walk. Find a pace that you can endure the entire time.

⑤

Immediate Count During and/or After an Aerobic Dance Routine

As you are beginning a conditioning aerobic dance program, you'll want to monitor your pace once or twice while you're learning a dance so that you can develop the skill of constant endurance pacing. This will lead up to your continual dancing for twenty-to-thirty, or more, minutes of the aerobic dance routines.

When you take a pulse rate during the learning process and find that your pace is **below** your established "training zone," do **more** work, or increase your intensity. If you are recording a pulse rate **higher** than your established "training zone," do **less** work, or lower your intensity. Continuing at a pace that is too intensive will prove to be an "anaerobic" exercise program — too much immediately followed by too little (you must recover and catch your breath). This yo-yo pace is **not** aerobic conditioning, so try for the constant pacing suggested previously.

The pulse monitoring procedure during aerobic dance is to slow down and walk, find your pulse, and count it for either **six, ten, or fifteen seconds.** Each of these counts has been found to be a scientifically accurate measurement for aerobic activity pulse rates. Once you (or your instructor) determine whether you will count for six, ten, or fifteen seconds **directly following aerobic dance, multiply the number you get times ten** if using the six-second count, **times six** if using a ten-second count, or **times four** if using a fifteen-second count. EACH OF THESE NEWLY MULTIPLIED NUMBERS WILL EQUAL HEARTBEATS PER MINUTE, and hopefully will be in your training zone!

NOTE: It is found to be easiest to take a six-second count, for all you do is "add a zero" to what pulse you feel and record that number. Persons must carefully begin and end exactly with a timer. Taking the immediate count during/after aerobic dance using a timed count of greater than fifteen seconds will tend to be inaccurate, since the heart rate slows down to a "recovery" pulse rather rapidly.

Also, you will soon recognize that as your cardiorespiratory system becomes more fit or efficient, work (exercise) will become easier, and you will be forced to increase the intensity of your activities by using larger arm movements, lifting your knees higher, hopping more, etc. By using the training zone, you automatically compensate for this increased fitness and still maintain the same training effect.

The count just mentioned is recorded as the "I", or immediate count taken during/after a dance and is recorded as such on the aforementioned chart. This count should **always** be in the training zone and doesn't fluctuate.

Since once you start and **never** completely stop or sit down until the latter part of the hour, **do not sit down to record** — simply bend over with a hamstring stretch, record, and keep walking. You do not want to encourage varicose veins, so keep moving!

Recovery Heart Rate Count, One Minute After

The recovery heart rate count, or "R" on the charting, is taken **one minute after** the previously monitored count (the "immediate" training zone count). This will visually show you on paper how your heart is recovering from strenuous exercise and is the **second measure of fitness that you can see happen on paper.** As you become more physically fit, the recovery count will get down lower and lower **away from** the immediate training zone count. This, then, is the reason for the count — so you can see your fitness improving on paper before your very eyes! It also provides a brief recovery interval to catch your breath for the **conditioning** dancer.

After the Cool-Down Exercise/Routine

This is only taken the first several weeks to show the new dancer how the heart responds to getting back to the pre-activity pulse count at which he or she started. This count should be **lower** than *120* beats per minute. Do not leave an hour or session of exercise with a higher heart rate. Lie on the floor another minute or two and retake the count until it comes down. Because you'll experience a concluding activity of relaxation, this count is eliminated after the first two weeks, and a count is taken only after relaxation at the end of the hour or session.

After Relaxation

In concluding the hour, a final count is taken to visually show the dancer several significant happenings. First, the heart rate may very well be **lower** than when the individual began the hour even with **only** three minutes of relaxation! And the individual will find that he or she, with a conscious effort to train the mind to relaxation, can get the heart rate down very close, if not to, each individual's **resting** heart rate!![3]

ENJOYMENT IS FOUND THROUGH VARIETY

Insure the success of this activity by having a program with variety and one in which you totally enjoy participating. Variety would include using all of the principles and possibilities in choreography (Chapter 8) and choosing a wide selection of music.

CHOOSE THE BEST LOCATION

Select a convenient and physiologically safe location for your program. Choose a **wood**-based floor or an area carpeted with flat nap and thick padding. Try not to exercise on concrete, since there is no "give" or buoyancy to it. Concrete adds unnecessary stress on your legs and feet.

SELECT PROPER CLOTHING TO WEAR

Choosing what to wear for the environment in which you are dancing is quite important. Comfort and ease of movement are the keys for aerobic dance apparel. Dress in layers. A warm-up sweatsuit or jogging suit will assist in increasing the temperature of your arm and leg muscles during the warm-up portion of the hour. On very warm, or highly humid and warm days, this, of course, is unnecessary. Select cotton material over others since it absorbs perspiration better than other fabrics. When cotton clothing becomes damp, the surrounding air causes the moisture to evaporate, and this will cool your body.

During the dance routines, you want to be free to move in all directions and sweat freely, so wear as little as possible when the temperature and relative humidity are high. Possibilities are shorts and a tee shirt, a leotard (and tights, but the tights **only** in cold weather), newly designed cotton exercise body suits, or — for women — shorts and a swimsuit with bra support for full-figured persons.

Wear proper-fitting cotton socks to help keep your feet free from blisters and to keep your feet drier. Underclothing needs to give you good support. Jockey shorts or, better yet, an athletic supporter for men and a bra that fits snugly and holds firmly for women, are important.

Just be sure that you do not wear too much clothing and get overheated. Persons very overweight or obese are especially prime targets for overheating because they have a thick layer of fat tissue between internal organs and the outside layer of skin. It works like insulation and keeps internal heat in. This means that the internal body systems may overheat and cause heat exhaustion or heat stroke. So don't try to "sweat" water pounds off by wearing lots of clothing or rubberlined sweatsuits. Sweat and water loss are your cooling mechanisms and are **not** to be used as a measurement for weight loss (for water is **not** fat!). A section on what **not** to wear is included in Chapter 11, "Special Concerns."

BUY THE PROPER SHOES

Appropriate, well-constructed shoes for this activity are a must! They will insure not only your comfort, but also will help prevent injuries (i.e., achilles tendon strain, heel bruises), particularly if all of this is new to you. You will find that this investment is well worth your attention — the dividends will pay off very soon after you begin your program. The following are guidelines when selecting an appropriate aerobic dance shoe. In order of importance:

YOUR AEROBIC DANCE PROGRAM

① Select a shoe that is designed to take the stress of repeated shock to the knees, lower legs, ankles, and feet. You **must** have a shoe that has a lot of cushioning in the arch and heel. In other words, wear a shoe with thick rubber soles!

② Do not select a wide heel flair (of rubber) if you have the tendency toward pronated ankles (lower leg bones do not sit directly on the ankle). This (heel flair) will not only limit, to some degree, your lateral (sideward) movement, but also it will not provide the appropriate correction to avoid future possible injury to naturally weak ankles, as it does in jogging — which is all forward movement. Pronation of ankles can best be corrected **inside** the shoe by means of:

- Raising the arch with a specifically designed wedge
- Bracing various portions of the foot by means of a specially designed orthotic (prescribed corrective device for the foot)
- An **extra firm** heel box

If you do not have pronated ankles, also purposefully select a rubber heel with no flair — one that is directly below the heel — to provide ease in executing the various sideward moves.

③ Try this on the shoe you're thinking of buying or using: bend the shoe in half (sole out) so that the toe is placed inside the heel. If the shoe bends, wear it. If the shoe doesn't bend very well, it will be an inflexible shoe in which

Figure 2.

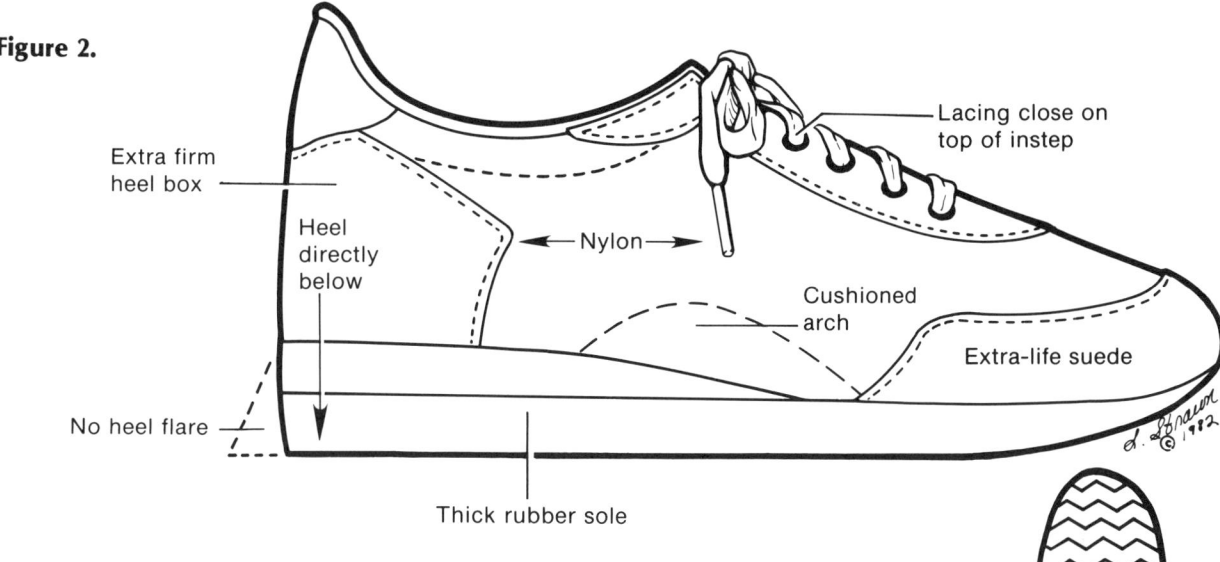

Pronated ankle (left) compared with a normal ankle (right).

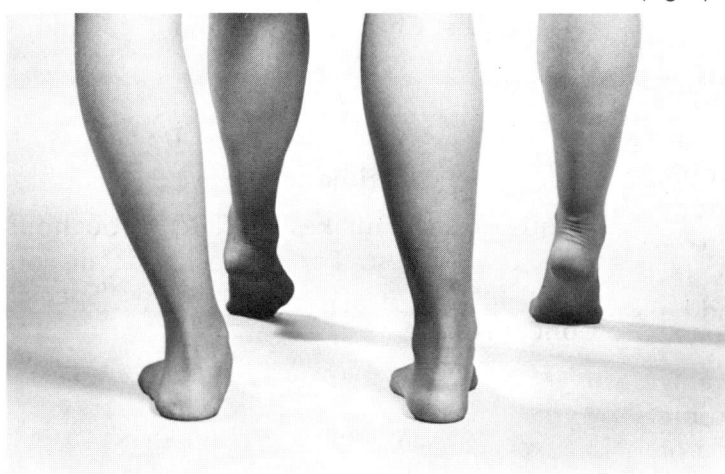

to dance. You want foot flexibility while you move.

④

Lacing should be of the style that has five or six eyelets **closely** spaced on the top of the instep. Wide lacing from the base of your toes across the entire instep will provide less support for lateral movement. This type of shoe ("low-tops") may tend to make your foot roll outward, causing ankle twisting or a sprain.

⑤

The sole of the shoe should have zig-zag lines that go from side to side and should be of white rubber, designed for court use. Jogging shoes with black rubber soles, designed for road and track running and with rubber triangles, squares, or circles or thick waves provide excellent **forward** movement, but since aerobic dance consists of forward, backward, and lateral movement, this is not a best first choice of shoe sole.

⑥

Nylon uppers are cooler than leather uppers. Extra design leather or suede along the ball-edge of the foot area (toes) provides for a longer shoe life.

Several companies are now making shoes that are specifically designed for aerobic dance. Any shoes that meet most of the above criteria should serve you well.

DEVELOP ASSOCIATED REGULAR HABITS: EATING/SLEEPING/RELAXING

In order to provide the fuel needed to produce the energy required for aerobic dance ("going"), and to insure proper body regulatory functions, growth, and repair ("growing"), eat a well-balanced diet that provides all the nutrients you need to stay well and be able to perform well (see Chapter 10).

Refrain from eating for one, or preferably two, hours before participating in aerobic activity. Eat afterwards. With the digestion of food, an increased amount of blood and oxygen is needed in the digestive tract. With exercise, as much as 100 times more oxygen is needed in the working muscles, i.e., arms and legs, than when at rest. Your body will just have great difficulty supplying an increase in blood and oxygen to two major body functions at once!

Establish quality time for proper relaxation and adequate sleep. These are important restorative mechanisms. Since aerobic dance will increase your energy level, the body's way of restoring energy ("energizing" you) is through relaxation and sleep. These also help to restore the ability to concentrate and to maintain a positive attitude and self-confidence. Physiologically, relaxation and sleep help by lowering both the body temperature and heart rate, which, in turn, lower the body's demand for oxygen and nutrients. These conserve, while restoring, the body's supply of energy.

INCORPORATE PROPER EXERCISE HABITS

①

Breathing Technique

Breathe continuously. Your entire system, especially your working muscles, **constantly need oxygen.** Holding your breath and turning red is **never** an appropriate way to exercise. While performing the warm-up and cool-down stretching (or any strengthening exercise), **exhale** when you **stretch,** and **inhale** when you **relax** your muscles. Cue yourself: "breathe out and stretch," breathe in and relax." (See Chapters 4, 6, and 7 for more specifics on breathing.)

②

Fluid Intake

Frequent small intakes of fluid throughout your day is best. For complete details on water intake, see Chapter 11 on "Special Concerns."

③

Missing a While?

Return to aerobic dance slowly. If for any

reason you miss activity several times, you will need to start more cautiously as though beginning a new program. For example, you may have a bout of flu and are then unable to exercise for a week. When you are able to exercise again, do **not** plan to start where you "left off." You will need to return cautiously to the fitness level that you were at before illness. Dr. Lenore Zohlman, a leading cardiologist in the United States, has stated that after just five weeks you will lose approximately half of your fitness program gains if you discontinue your program totally. And, after ten weeks of no aerobic activity, you will have lost most of the fitness gains that you experienced.[4] So realize this physiological phenomenon and return slowly and systematically whenever a circumstance curtails your program.

CONSIDER THE VARIABLES

There are numerous variables to be considered and planned for when engaging in an aerobic dance program. A few are:

- The environmental temperature
- The relative humidity
- Physiological changes with the menstrual cycle
- Illness, infection, or injury present
- The amount of negative stress you are currently experiencing

All of these variables will make changes in how your body responds during an aerobic dance program. Be flexible in your program when any new factor enters into the picture and change your procedure accordingly.

①

Above 85° F. room or outside temperature, never aerobic dance — go aerobic swim in an air-conditioned environment.

②

A high relative humidity combined with a hot day are two good reasons to, again, aerobic swim in an air-conditioned environment. (You can develop heat stress even in an outside pool in a hot and humid environment. The key is the **cool** air temperature.)

③

For many women, the menstrual cycle creates no new concerns. Practicing good habits of physical fitness and nutrition[5] are the best words of advice to alleviate any temporary discomforts experienced. (Refer to Chapter 11, "Special Concerns," for more details.)

④

The presence of illness, infection, or injury will show up in your "thermometer" of fitness — your pulse. It will be higher at rest and will escalate to the training zone with less than your usual effort. So take it easy and decide whether to mentally "walk" through your program to maintain your discipline of exercising, or to just curtail exercise until you're well again.

⑤

Negative stress, like illness, will escalate your heart rate **at rest or during aerobic dancing.** You, again, will have to closely monitor your heart rate to keep it at your training zone so that you don't overtax your heart. (More on stress-related information in Chapter 7.)

Other varibles to be considered are the presence of various temporary limitations, or injury-related concerns. A complete discussion can be found in Chapter 11.

AEROBIC DANCE — A NEW RELEASE FROM STRESS

Because we are all victims of unwanted daily pressures, we all find a way to release these pressures. Some ways are good for our health and some are detrimental. But what we must recognize is that we all do **something** to release the stress and tensions in our lives! It is the way we maintain our mental balance — the way in which we cope with life. Some people smoke, some drink alcohol, or coffee, or soda pop to excess, others eat to excess,

22 YOUR AEROBIC DANCE PROGRAM

some play loud music or bang out a few tunes on a musical instrument, some chew gum wildly — the list is endless! Some habits are harmless; some are harmful.

If you don't like the way you look and feel — if you're too fat, too lean and weak, too out of breath doing any daily activities, are listless, or bored, then try allowing aerobic dance to assist you in alleviating that unwanted stress. Using aerobic dance as your **stress release** will give you a healthy outlet for all those problems or situations or pressures that you accumulate. You can get so turned on to aerobic dance that at the end of a session, you can pick up those cares that you put aside for a few moments and charge into them with renewed vigor! Life is situations and life is change. How we each adapt to and cope with these situations or changes reveals our true human quality. So, forget all those unhealthy crutches you've established as **habits of choice** to relieve the stress in your life!

Smoking

Smoking tobacco causes the lung capillaries to decrease in size (constrict), which, in turn, restricts the ability of your cardiorespiratory system to circulate the needed oxygen to your body parts. When you are performing an activity that requires the use of more oxygen, why would you want to compound the situation by **choosing** to allow less oxygen supply and use to take place?

Alcohol

Try to abstain from the use of the number one drug problem — alcohol. Alcohol causes a constriction of the coronary arteries supplying the heart at the same time your exercise program is demanding an **increase** of oxygen from the heart. Again, why **choose** to allow less oxygen and nutrient supply to occur when you need more? Kick the habit and get "hooked" on aerobic dance instead. If you do drink, do so in moderation after exercising or at least four hours before you aerobic dance. And then work at a decreased intensity level. The two activities — drinking followed by aerobic dancing — simply do not go together.

Overeating

Consuming far too much food is a habit by **choice** that all too many Americans engage in today. Chapter 9 contains quite an extensive discussion on this topic, since it is one of the **primary** reasons why people begin aerobic dancing.[6]

EVALUATE YOUR PROGRESS AND PROGRAM

Review the monitored data you've been collecting on yourself. It may seem quite remarkable how one fun-filled activity can create so much positive change for the better in most individuals.

A REVIEW CHECKLIST

Go through the following to be sure you've tryed your best to plan and execute a top-notch program for yourself.

- Assess fitness in the very beginning
- Set realistic goals
- Plan time on a weekly basis
- Develop your skill at pulse taking
- Chart your progress:
  - Monitoring resting pulse rate
  - Monitoring various segments of the aerobic dance session
  - Weight maintenance/loss/gain
  - Dietary intake
  - Journal on mental and emotional change
- Enjoyment is found through variety
- Choose the best location
- Select proper clothing to wear
- Buy the proper shoes for this unique activity
- Develop associated regular habits: Eating/Sleeping/Relaxing
- Incorporate proper exercise habits: Breathing Technique/Fluid Intake/Missing Activity/and Beginning Again
- Consider the variables: Temperature/Rela-

tive Humidity/Menstrual Cycle/Illness, Infection, or Injury/Presence of Negative Stress
- Allow aerobic dance to become your new release from stress: Forget Smoking/Alcohol/Overeating
- Evaluate your progress and your program

KEEP DANCING — KEEP SMILING — KEEP FIT

You have completed your aerobic dance program preparation, and now you are ready to begin! Dr. George Sheehan, author of numerous running articles and books, states that aerobic dance is on target, helping one's fitness, as well as helping one psychologically. Many people who have been habitual dropouts from other fitness programs are now enthusiastic and dedicated members of aerobic dance programs. The combination of music, dance, and the social atmosphere can become irresistible.

We hope that you will consider aerobic dance so much fun and so beneficial that you'll be involved for life!

3

POSTURE: WHERE IT ALL BEGINS

A requisite to aerobic dance and to life itself is good posture. Proper posture is the basis for effective movement patterns. Good posture means aligning the skeletal system to lessen the friction of bone against bone and to prevent muscles from shortening and rubbing against each other — thus alleviating muscular aches and pains.

The word "posture" means position. You have many postures or positions throughout your daily living. There are two kinds: (1) **static** (still) posture, used to understand correct postural techniques; and (2) **dynamic** (moving) posture, which is the kind almost always in use. When you have correct posture, your body is in a balanced position. This involves distributing your weight in a balanced way from the front of your body to the back and from side to side.

ESTABLISHING GOOD POSTURE

As you develop good postural awareness, you will move in well-aligned positions. An efficient position is one in which the various body segments are balanced above each other so that there is a minimum of friction and uneven pressure in the weight-bearing joints and a minimum of strain on muscles and ligaments. This enables a margin of safety in each joint so that no unexpected force can push the joint beyond its normal limits and cause injury. When your body is in proper alignment, it is in the best position to resist the downward pull of gravity with the least amount of stress and effort.

Good posture is best maintained by having:

①

The head and stretched neck balanced on top of the spine and centered above the shoulders, keeping your chin parallel to the floor.

②

Your shoulders pulled back and down (in a relaxed position).

③

Your chest and rib cage raised up.

POSTURE: WHERE IT ALL BEGINS

④

Your abdominal muscles pulled in and up under the rib cage.

⑤

The pelvic girdle pulled down and under, tightening the gluteal muscles. The pelvis rests on the two thigh bones balanced over two arched feet.

⑥

Your knees relaxed. Locking your knees in a hyperextended position causes imbalance and makes you more susceptible to knee injury.

⑦

Your weight distributed equally on both feet while standing with feet parallel and toes pointing forward as you take the weight on the outer edges of the feet.

⑧

Your arms relaxed.

If any segment is out of body alignment, your weight distribution is uneven over your base of support and puts unnecessary strain on muscles, bones, and joints. This causes fatigue.

Postural problems are caused by muscular imbalance, and muscular imbalance is caused by habitual positions and environmental conditions that establish inefficient movement patterns. For example, the muscles in the calves of your legs will be shortened if you wear high heels frequently. Most muscles are in pairs, so if a muscle shortens, its opposing muscle will lengthen and become weak from disuse. Stretching one set of muscles and strengthening the opposing set of muscles will improve your posture.

To have erect posture, the position of the hip joints (which act as the main hinges of the body) and of the pelvic girdle needs to be controlled primarily by strong abdominal and gluteal muscles. The anti-gravity muscle groups that hold us erect are located in the calves, in front of our thighs, in the back along the spinal column, in the buttocks, and in the abdomen. In order to have good posture, these muscles need to be strong enough to perform their function and relaxed enough to perform with ease. Each joint needs to be flexible enough to permit a full range of movement. A kinesthetic awareness needs to be developed so that you feel uncomfortable when moving through tasks incorrectly or inefficiently. For example, having strength and flexibility in the lower back, hip, and thigh areas makes it possible to have balanced pelvic alignment. And if the front of your thighs are strong, you can stoop, sit, and walk up and down stairs more efficiently.

EFFICIENT BASIC POSTURE PATTERNS

Correct posture and movement patterns as you sit, stand, walk, and move about doing daily tasks will help you strengthen the muscles needed to keep the body in good alignment. This is the **best** exercise that you can do for yourself — to be aware of good postural principles with every move you make. For example:

①

An important rule for good posture while sitting is to have your knees higher than your hips; otherwise, the back tends to overarch.

②

Standing can tire the back. Solve this by elevating a foot. This flexes one hip and keeps the lower back from straining forward. For example, when standing at the sink doing dishes, open the cupboard door underneath the sink and rest one foot on the ledge. Try it. Feel the difference?

A standing position requires more energy to maintain balance than sitting or lying positions. Remember — the broader your base of support, the lower the center of gravity, allowing for better balance. (Regardless what posture you are assuming, always apply this principle for greater efficiency of movement.)

26 POSTURE: WHERE IT ALL BEGINS

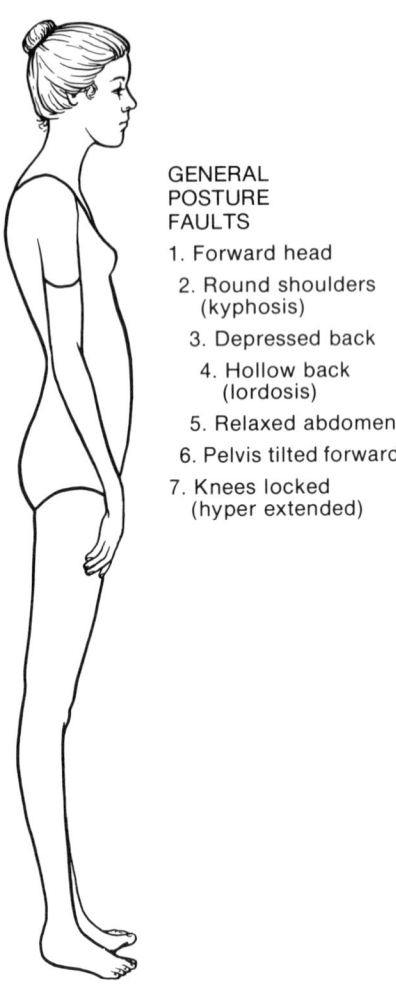
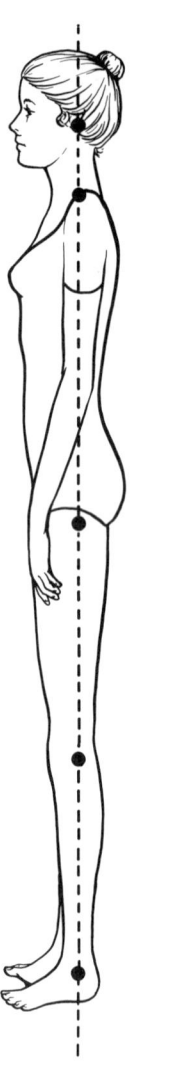
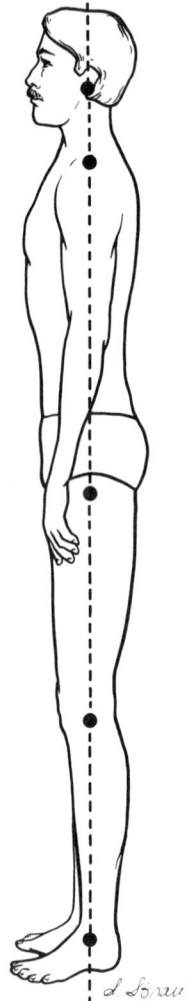

GENERAL POSTURE FAULTS
1. Forward head
2. Round shoulders (kyphosis)
3. Depressed back
4. Hollow back (lordosis)
5. Relaxed abdomen
6. Pelvis tilted forward
7. Knees locked (hyper extended)

BALANCED STANDING POSTURE
1. Chin parallel to floor
2. Ear above middle of shoulder
3. Tip of shoulder over hip joint
4. Shoulders relaxed and down
5. Chest and rib cage lifted
6. Front of pelvis and thigh in a continuous line
7. Knees unlocked or slightly flexed
8. Feet parallel, body weight centered between heel and toe

Figure 3.

To lessen unnecessary strain on the back while sleeping, lie on your side with your hips and knees bent and your head supported by a pillow.

WHAT GOOD POSTURE DOES FOR YOU

Posture is an important factor in the impression you make on others and in your feelings of well-being and self-confidence. Good posture improves your appearance, helps give confidence, promotes better health, allows the organs room to function properly, and lessens the possibility of accidental injury. In other words, correct body alignment has a direct influence on your comfort and work efficiency and on your coordination. The poise that comes with good posture projects an image of positive thinking and shows that you feel good about yourself.

POSTURE — A HABIT TO BE CHANGED

Posture is definitely a habit that can be changed, but it will take time, since the habit that you now have has been a part of you for a long time. You need to re-educate your neuromuscular system, and this will take understanding, persistence, and a sincere desire on your part to improve both your appearance and the efficiency of your body. If your body is to move freely, every muscle needs to be able to relax and lengthen as well as be able to contract strongly and quickly. Exercises in Chapters 4 and 6 have a threefold purpose. They help you to warm up and cool down as they improve your posture by stretching and strengthening anti-gravity muscle groups. Remember — time spent on posture exercises is just a **small** part of bringing about posture change.

Balanced posture makes full and efficient use of the force of gravity by aligning all parts so that the pull is directly downward through the supporting parts. This allows the muscles to do minimal work in maintaining the body in an erect position. The ligaments and muscles surrounding each joint hold the part in place, cooperating with the pull of gravity instead of constantly having to work against it. Efficiency is obtained, since the less work muscles have to do, the less energy they expend and the less fatigue they experience.

IN SUMMARY

Good posture is established by persistent practice. Start now. Are you sitting correctly? As you practice good habitual posture, there is less strain on the back muscles and less fatigue. Being constantly aware of good posture — standing tall and pulling your abdomen up and in with your rib cage lifted, making your torso erect — is the best **one** exercise that you can do.

The knowledge of a well-aligned body and the kinesthetic awareness (feeling) of good posture are the first steps in acquiring good posture habits. Practicing on a daily basis is required for good posture to become a reality.

Remember:

- Stand with your weight distributed equally on both feet
- Keep knees easy
- Pull pelvic girdle down and under as you tighten buttocks
- Raise your ribs **up** from your hips
- Pull your abdomen in and up under the ribs
- Pull your shoulders back and down in a relaxed position
- Stretch your neck **up** from your shoulders
- Place your head in alignment with your spine, with your chin parallel to the floor
- Keep your arms relaxed

When exercising, moving efficiently and effectively depends on proper body alignment. Think good posture at all times. Improve while you move all day, every day.

4

WARM-UPS: EXERCISES AND ROUTINES

FUNCTION OF THE WARM-UP

The warm-up period is important to help assure a safe and comfortable aerobic dance program. Its function is to help the muscles prepare for the stresses of vigorous activity by increasing the blood flow to muscles and connective tissues. As the blood vessels in the muscles dilate and the tendons and ligaments are stretched, the muscles become more supple and relaxed. This makes them less likely to be strained or torn by strenuous activity.

The warm-up period prepares the body to meet the increased demand for oxygen needed by the heart, lungs, and muscles during vigorous activity. **All** parts of the body need to be warmed up before the aerobic dance phase of your program. Warming up completely before **every** workout is a wise habit to develop. Not only does it prepare you physically, it also prepares you mentally for the strenuous workout in which you are engaging.

The biggest danger in starting a strenuous activity without a warm-up is the possibility of tearing or pulling a muscle. It's especially important for people over the age of thirty to warm up, since some flexibility may have been lost. This is the reason why stretching and flexibility exercises that loosen the muscles are good to do before aerobic dance. The time needed for a complete warm-up varies with the individual, since each person is at a different level of fitness. A good guideline would be a **minimum** of five to ten minutes of warm-up exercises.

FLEXIBILITY DEVELOPED BY STRETCHING

A good rule to follow is to warm up with activities related to the activity in which you wish to participate. For example, if you are aerobic dancing, begin with a slower tempoed, easy-moving dance, and then increase the tempo or speed and the intensity of the movement patterns. The warming up period

WARM-UPS: EXERCISES AND ROUTINES

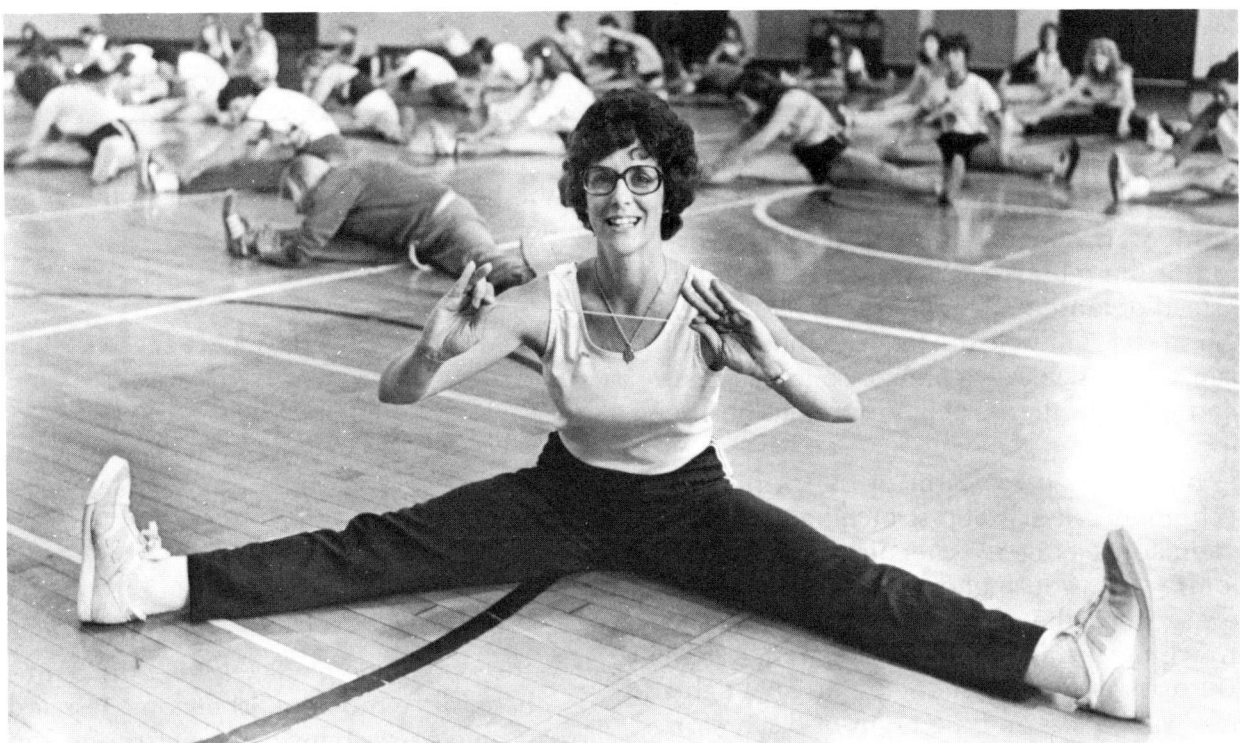

FLEXIBILITY TRAINING IS ACHIEVED THROUGH STRETCHING
Your muscles are like rubberbands. They remain relaxed if no pull is exerted on either end. If one end of a rubberband or muscle is slowly moved away from a stationary point (joint), however, the rubberband or muscle slowly stretches, or lengthens. With numerous repetitions, each will become warmer. As the end of either is relaxed again and allowed to return to its original position, the muscle shortens, or contracts.

Improper stretching will cause pain and physical damage due to microscopic tearing of minute muscle fibers. This leads to the formation of scar tissue in the muscle, with gradual loss of elasticity.

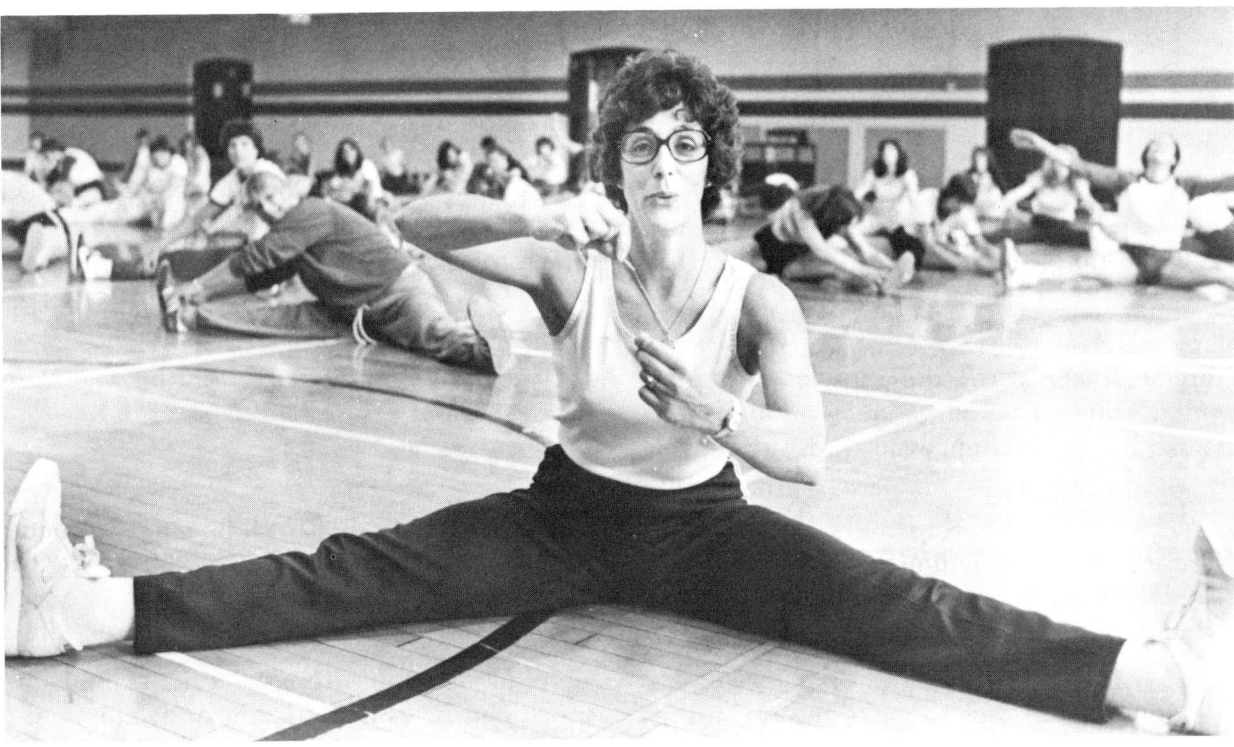

is also a good opportunity to increase your flexibility.

The key to executing the warm-up exercises efficiently is to ease gently into a **stretched** position and hold it as you press. Push to the point of tightness (**not** pain) so that you feel the muscles working. Bouncing or jerking during warm-up may cause a reflex contraction of the muscles, which increases tension instead of loosening the muscle fibers. When you stretch a muscle too far or to the point of pain, the muscle will tighten or contract rather than increase the flexibility or range of motion.

The best way to warm up is to utilize a technique called static stretching. This is a gradual reaching in one direction. At the point where you feel discomfort, hold for a few seconds, then slowly withdraw and begin stretching in the opposite direction. When you repeat the first action, the original tightness will be less and the point of discomfort will move farther away as you become more flexible.

Slowly stretching and pressing the muscles make them more supple, which allows greater ease of movement. As you increase the intensity of the exercise slowly, your body begins to feel loose, warm, and ready for the rigorous activity of aerobic dance. It not only increases your flexibility, it also helps in reducing tension.

The warm-up sequence of exercises needs to be designed with the following components:

①

A gradual increase in intensity of exercise as the warm-up progresses.

②

Exercises that stretch the muscles and put joints through a whole range of motion but that do not strain them against resistance.

③

Exercises that are rhythmic in nature with a natural flow from one to the next.

④

A variety of exercises to make the warm-up enjoyable.

⑤

A combination of muscle stretching with increased activity of the cardiovascular system.

⑥

All body segments and natural motions included.

POINTS TO REMEMBER

When warming up for an aerobic dance workout, remember to:

①

Warm up the **entire** body.

②

Start the workout immediately after the warm-up phase, since the benefits become less and less as time passes between the warm-up and the workout.

CONTROLLED BREATHING

While exercising and/or dancing, it is important to breathe rhythmically. Do not hold your breath. Proper breathing helps to facilitate the delivery of extra oxygen to the working muscles. When executing the stretching and pressing exercises, exhale as you stretch and press, and inhale with each recovery or relaxation of the muscle.

THREEFOLD PURPOSE

The following exercises will help to:

①

Warm up the body parts for the vigorous dances.

②

Cool down the body parts following the dance workout.

③

Help to develop strength and flexibility in specific muscles for efficient body alignment (improved posture).

1
Shoulder Shrug

(Upper back and shoulders)

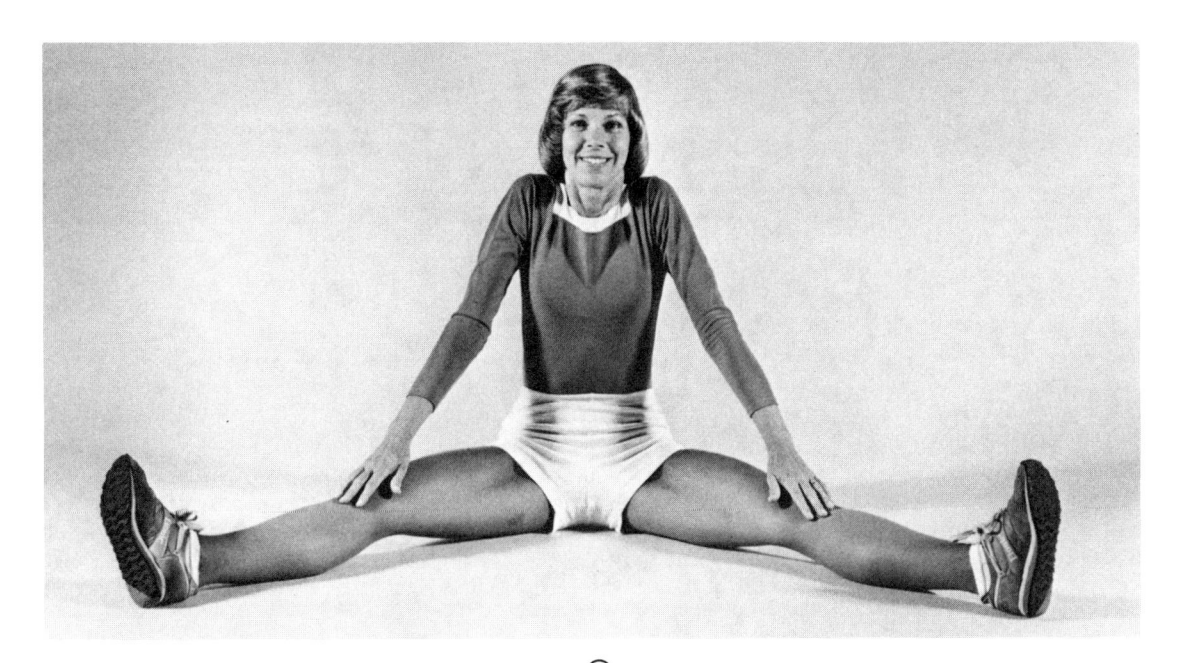

①
Sit in a widestride position, keeping the back and legs straight and arms at the sides of the body. Lift your shoulders directly upward as high as possible. Hold.

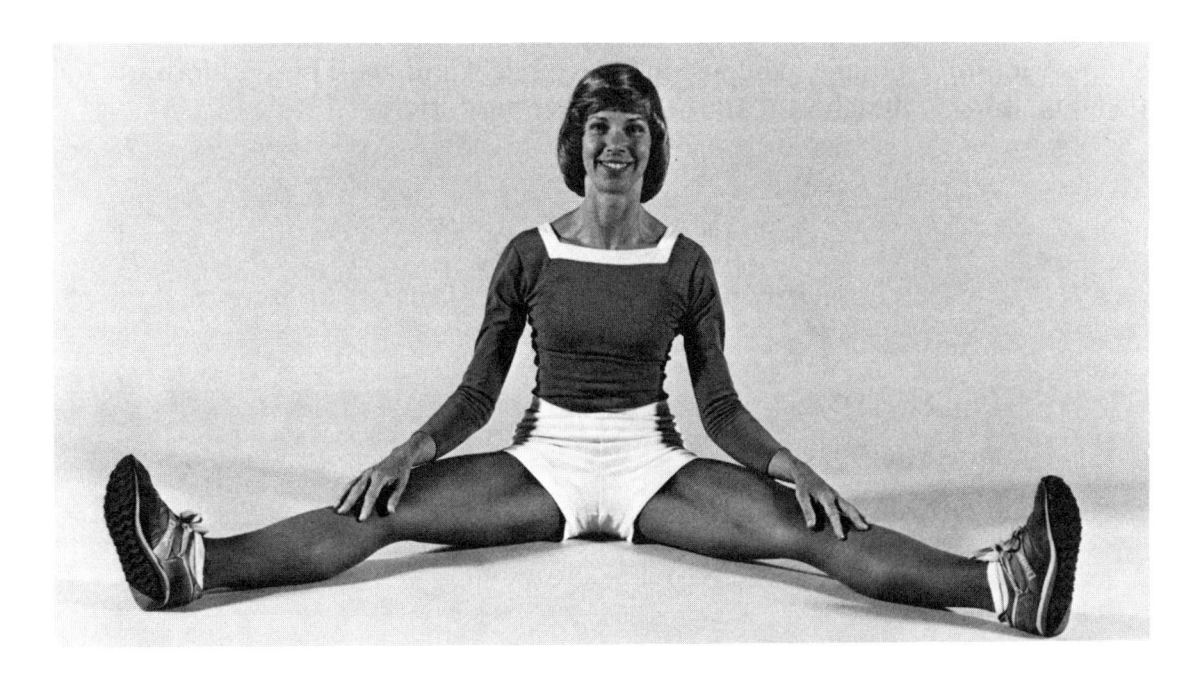

②
Lower your shoulders pressing downward. Hold.

2
Widestride Press

(Lower back and back of leg)

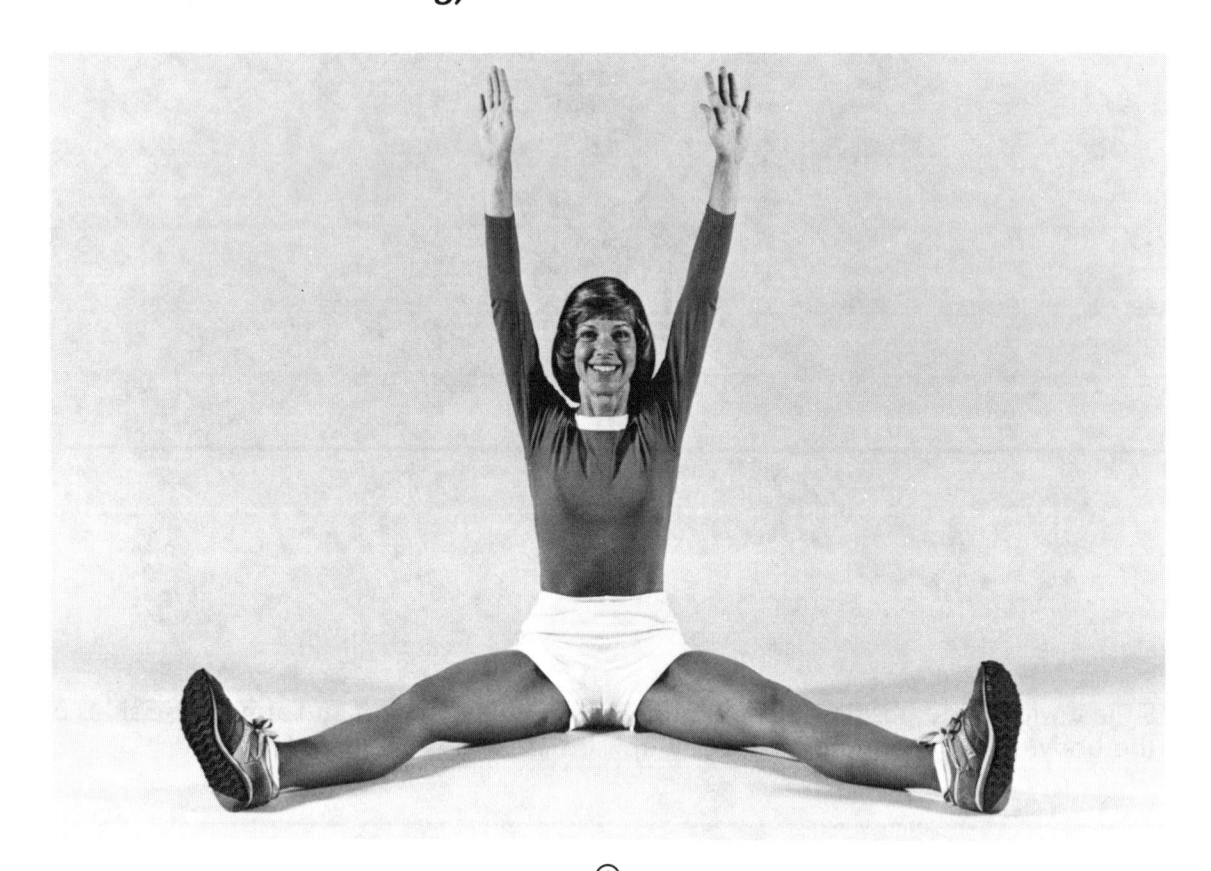

①
Sit in a widestride position, keeping the legs straight and heels pressed forward, toes pointing upward. Stretch your arms above your head. Hold.

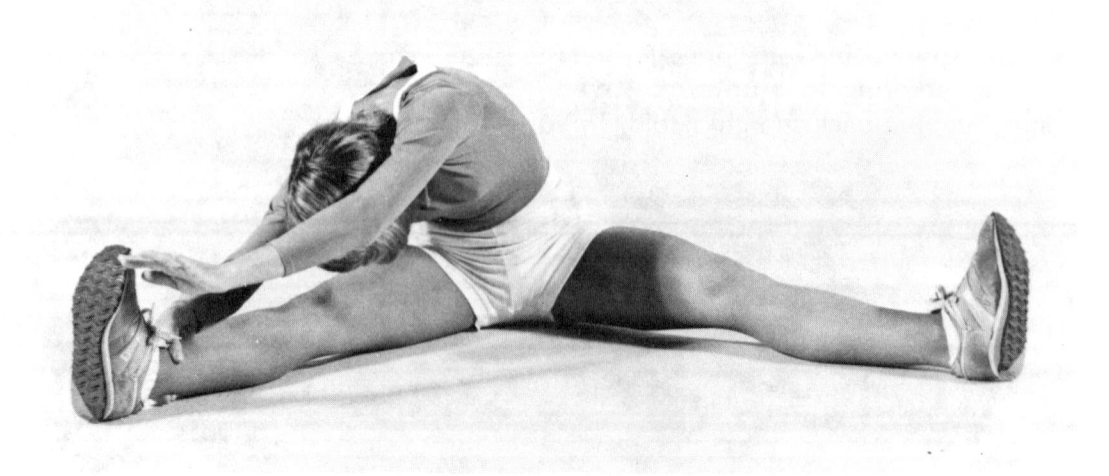

②
Turn the upper body toward the right leg, and bend forward slowly at the hip, grasping as far down the leg as possible. Press the head as close to the knee as possible. Hold.

WARM-UPS: EXERCISES AND ROUTINES   33

③
Return to starting position described in ①. Hold.

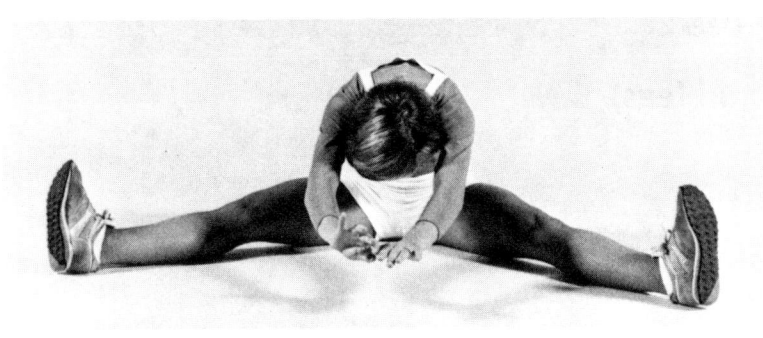

④
Facing front, bend forward slowly at the hips, stretching the arms in front. Stretch forward and press downward, leading with the chin. Hold.

⑤
Return to position ①. Hold.

⑥
Turn the upper body toward the left leg, and bend forward slowly at the hip, grasping (but not pulling) as far down the leg as possible. Press the head as close to the knee as possible. Hold.

⑦
Return to position ①. Hold.

⑧
Repeat ④. Hold.

⑨
Return to position ①. Hold.

3
Legs In Front Press

(Back and legs)

①
Sit with legs straight in front, pressing heels forward and pointing toes upward. Stretch arms high, keeping back straight. Hold.

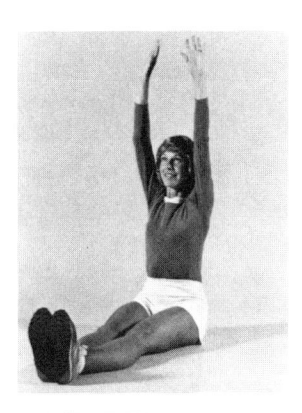

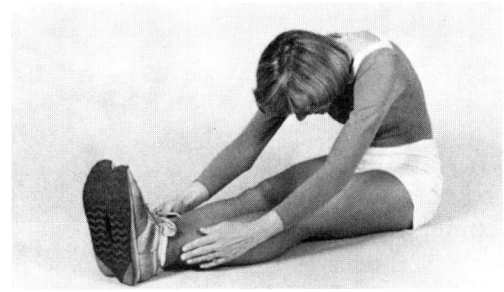

②
Slowly reach as far forward as possible, pressing the upper body downward with the top of the head toward the feet. Keep legs straight. Hold.

4
Widestride Hug
(Waist, midriff, and legs)

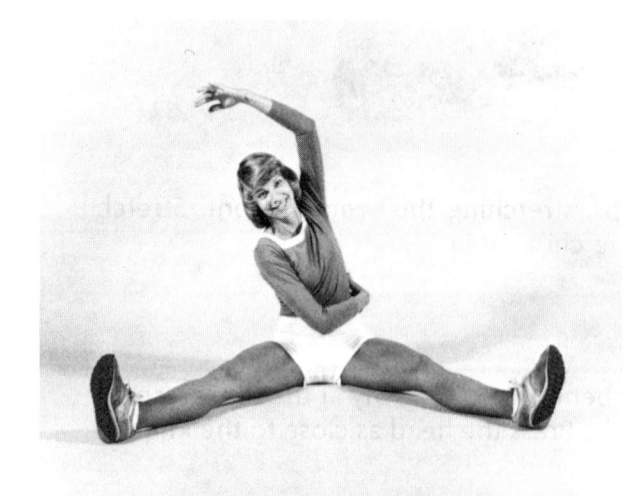

①
Sit in a widestride position, keeping the legs straight. Wrap your right arm around your waist, and turn the upper body diagonally to the left. Bring the left arm curved over the head to the right side.

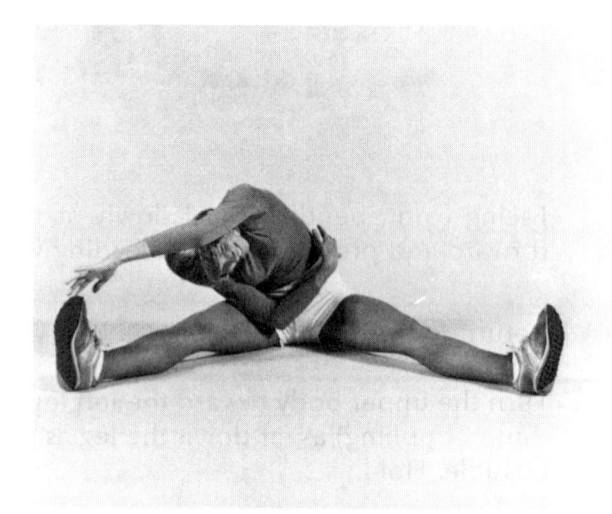

②
Slowly press the right side of the head as close as possible to the right knee, bringing the left hand as close as possible to the right foot. Press and hold.

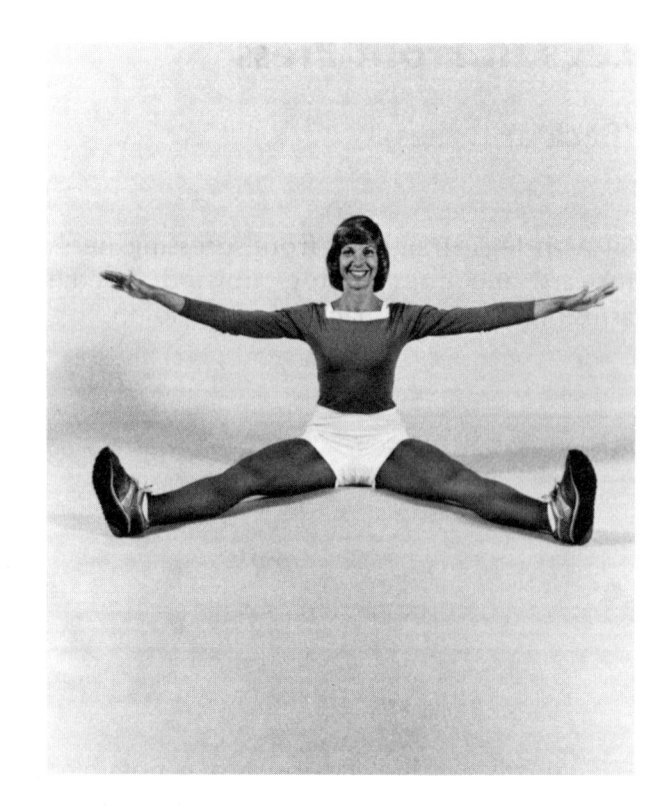

③
Sit tall in a widestride position with the back straight, heels pressing forward, toes pointing upward, and arms stretched straight out from the shoulders. Hold.

④
Repeat, pressing to the left side. Hold.

WARM-UPS: EXERCISES AND ROUTINES 35

5
Lateral Bend

(Trunk and waist)

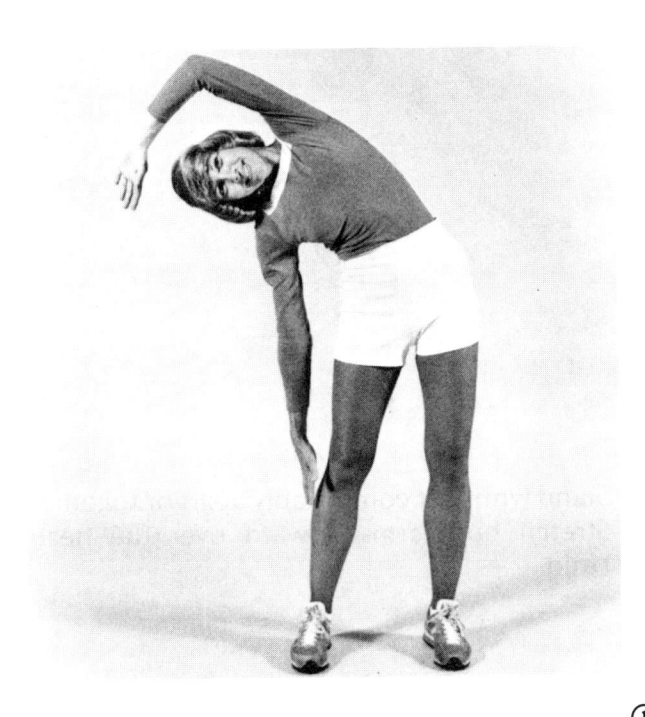

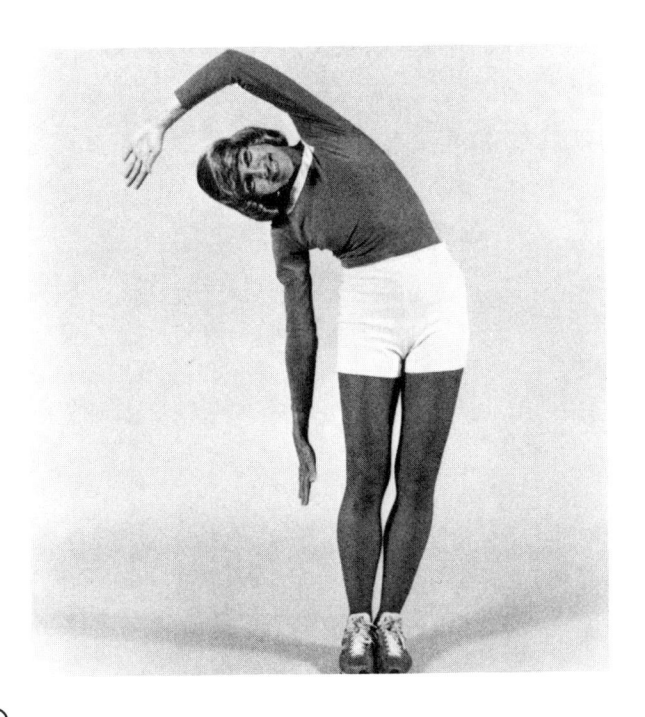

①
Stand with good posture. Feet can be shoulder-width apart (left) or placed side by side (right). Keep legs straight. Right arm is dropped to the side of the body. Raise the left arm upward over your head. With chest high, abdomen pulled in, and buttocks firm, bend trunk and left arm to the side as far as possible. Hold.

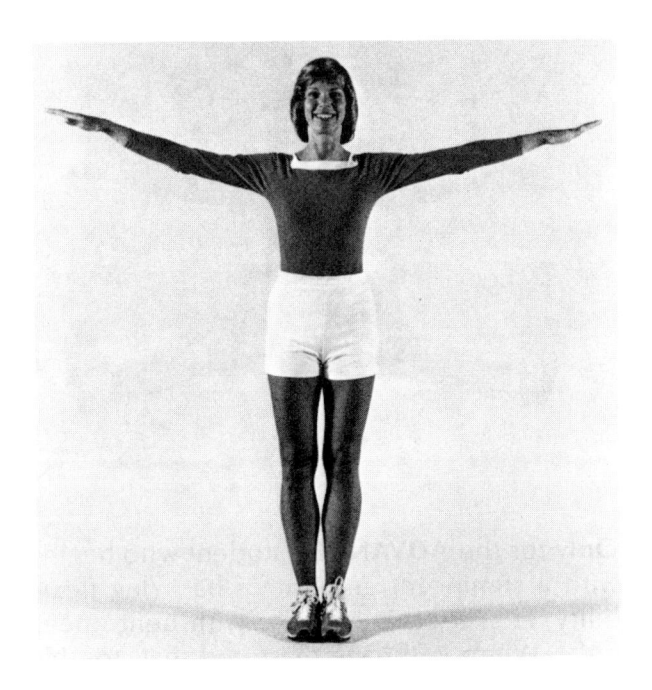

②
Stand tall in a stretched position with the arms straight out from the shoulders. Hold.

③
Bend laterally to the left side. Hold.

④
Repeat ②. Hold.

36 WARM-UPS: EXERCISES AND ROUTINES

6

Front Toe Touch

(Back and legs)

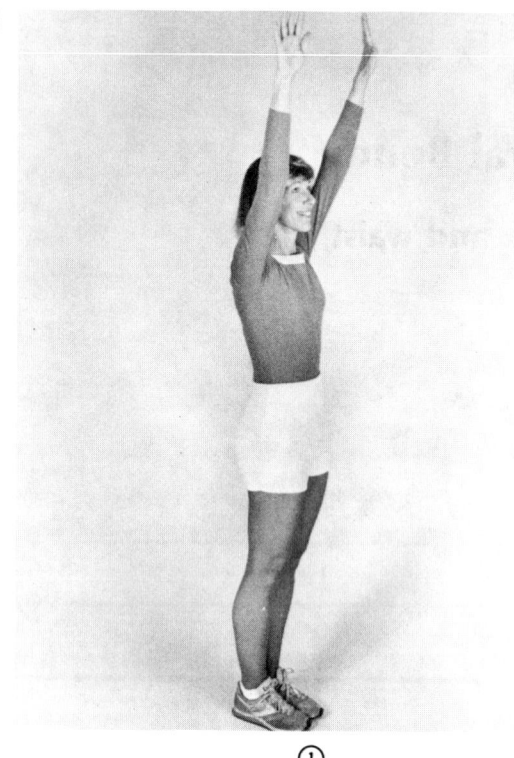

①
Stand with feet comfortably apart or together. Stretch both arms upward over the head. Hold.

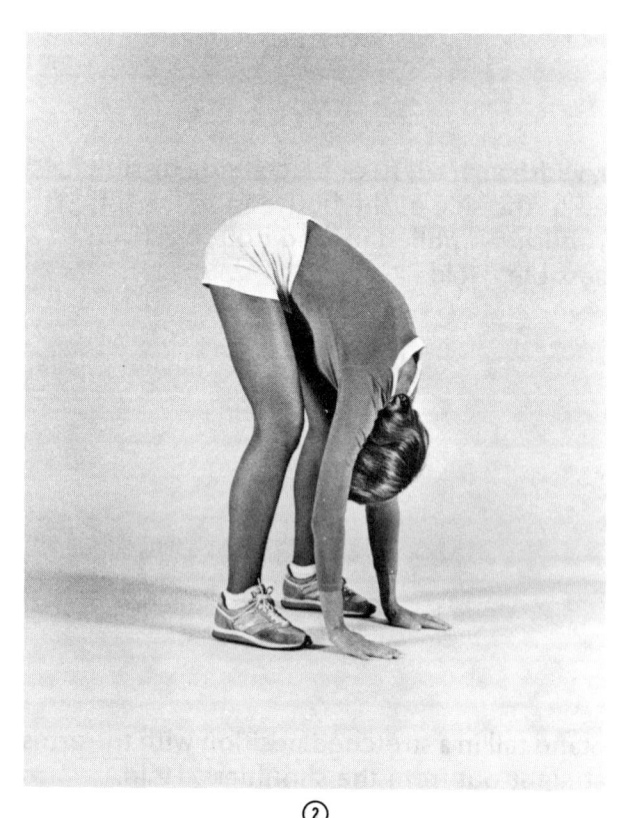

②
Bend trunk and arms forward and downward. Stretch **slowly** and gently, bending the knees and placing palms on the floor. Head should be relaxed downward, with the top of your head toward the floor. Hold.

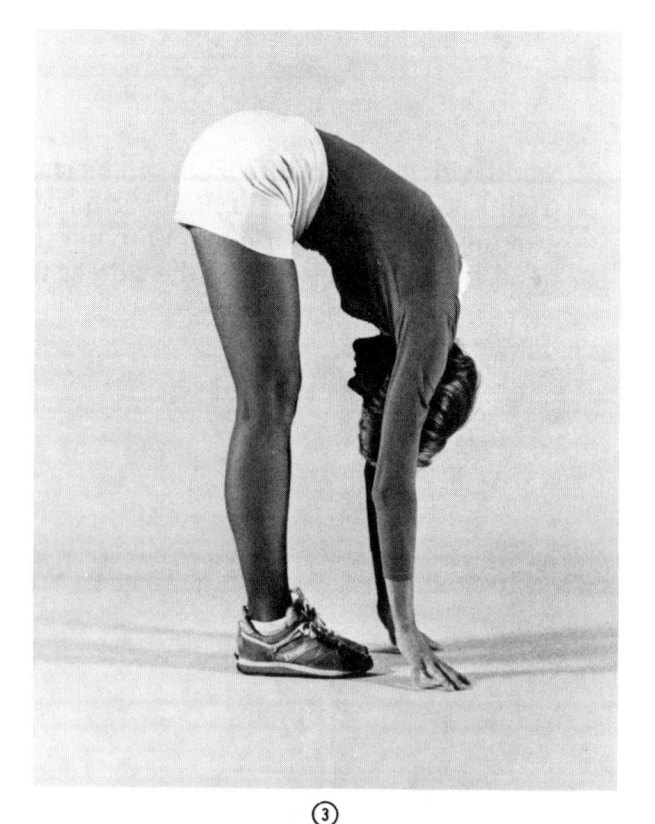

③
Only for the **ADVANCED** student who begins with a significant amount of back/leg flexibility. First try this exercise with bent knees (left). When you have mastered that, try this exercise with the legs straight **without** locking the knees (right).

7
Knee Lift
(Back and hips)

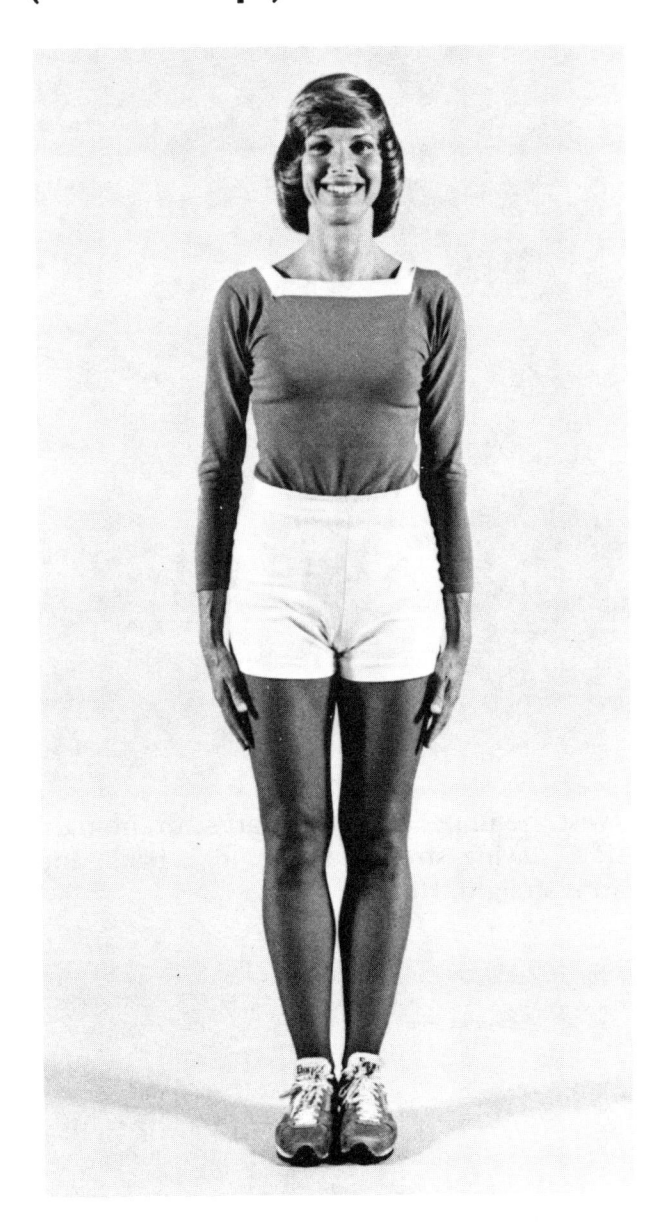

①
Stand erect with feet together and arms at sides.

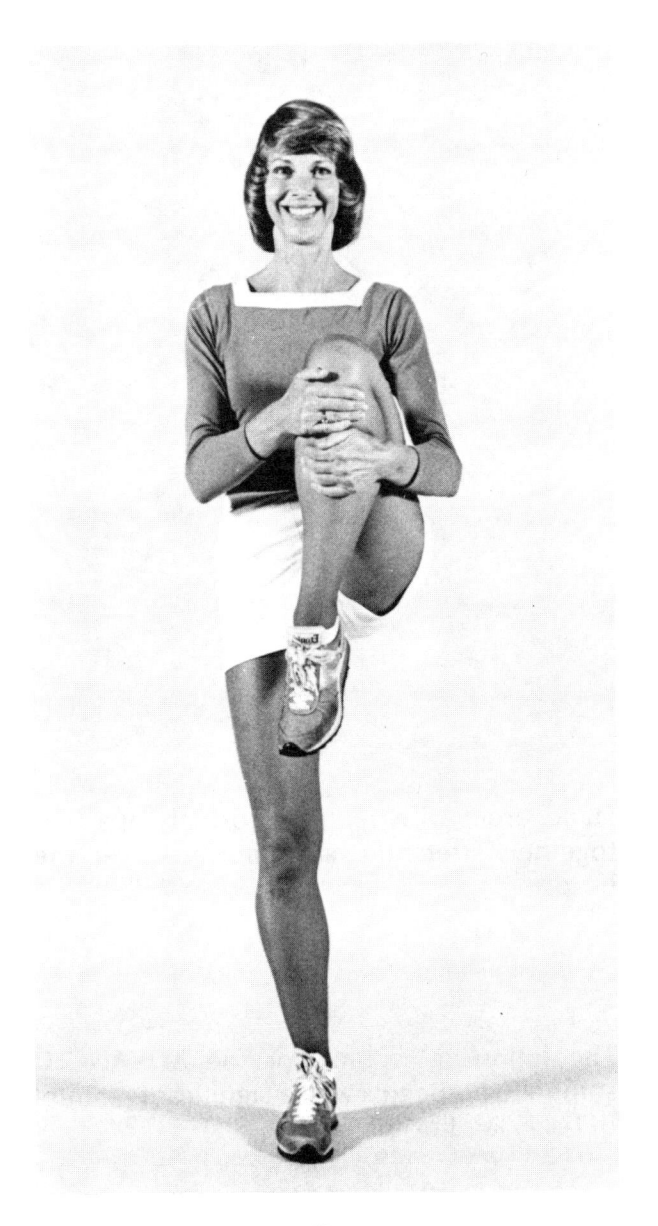

②
Raise left knee as high as possible, grasping the leg with both hands and pulling the knee against the chest while keeping the back straight. Hold. Can rotate ankle/foot joints.

③
Repeat ①.

④
Repeat ②, lifting the right knee. Hold.

8
Twisting Toe Touch
(Trunk, arms, and legs)

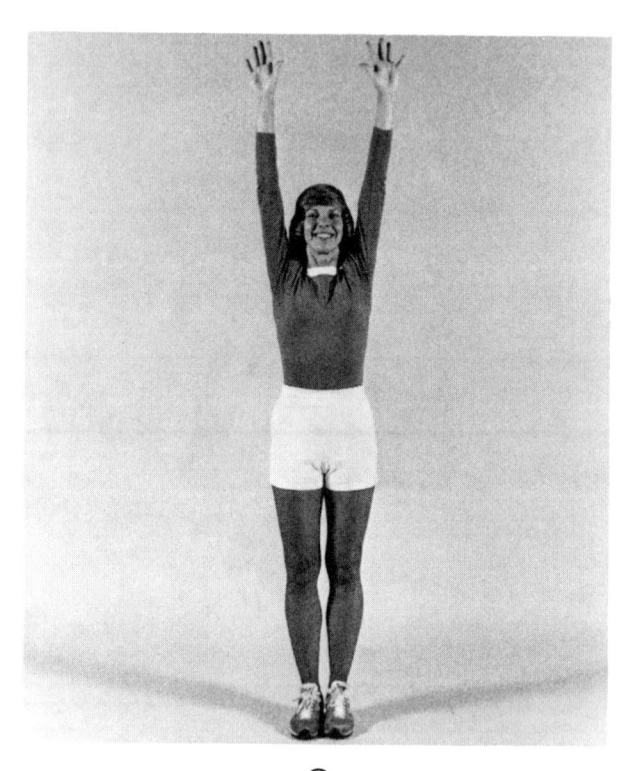

①
Stand erect with feet comfortably apart or together, stretching arms upward over the head.

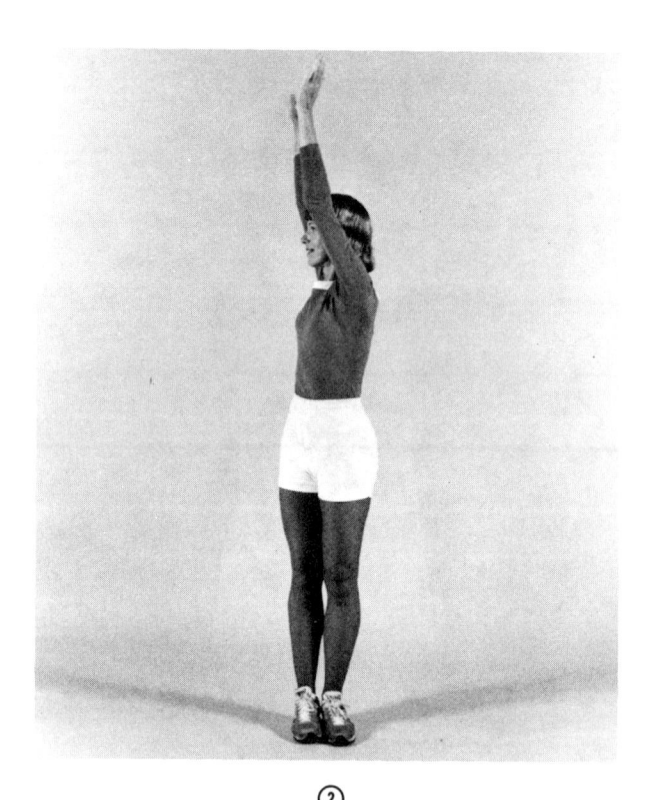

②
Twist the upper body 90 degrees to the right side, staying stretched with legs, back, and arms straight. Hold.

The following is only for the **ADVANCED** student who begins with a significant amount of back/leg flexibility.

③
Bend trunk and arms downward as far as possible, bringing the nose toward the knees and keeping the legs straight, knees slightly flexed.

④
Return to position ②.

⑤
Return to position ①.

⑥
Repeat this exercise to the left side.

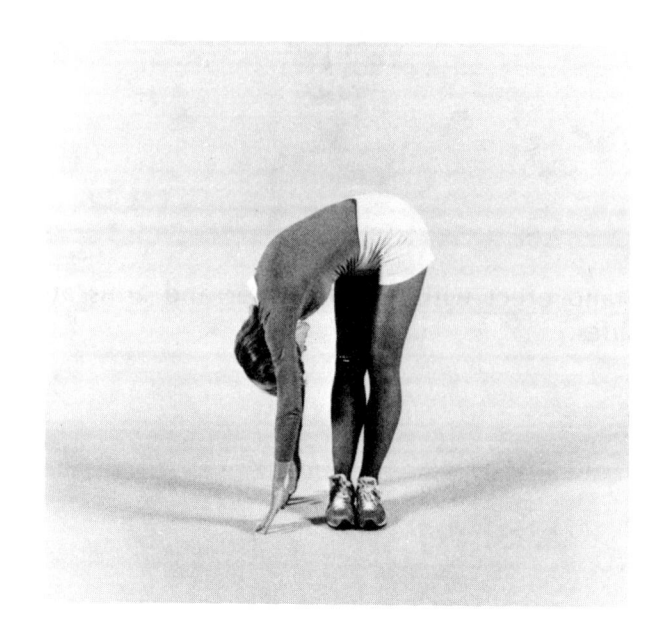

9
Front Lunge

(Legs and buttocks)

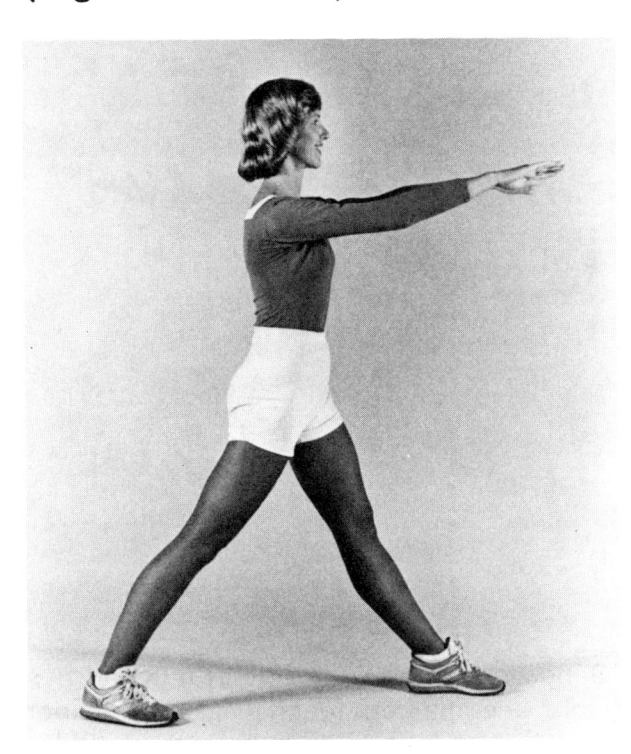

①
Stand in a wide stance position with one foot in front of the body and the other foot in back of the body. Keep the hips squared, facing front. The arms are in front at shoulder level to help maintain balance. Point both feet forward.

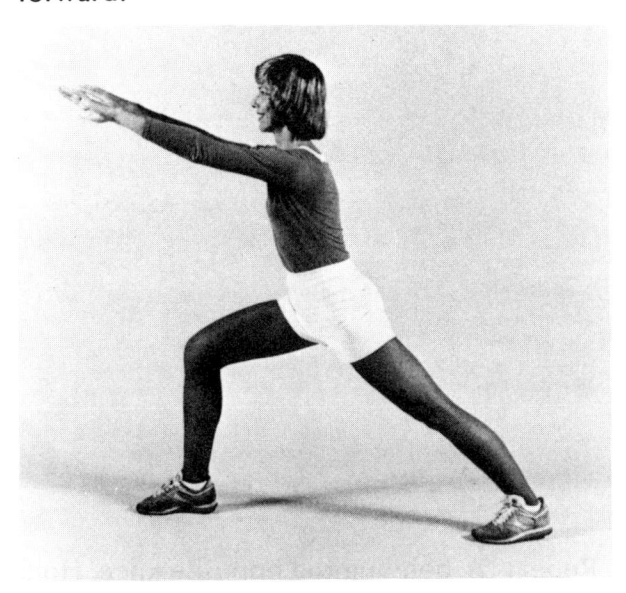

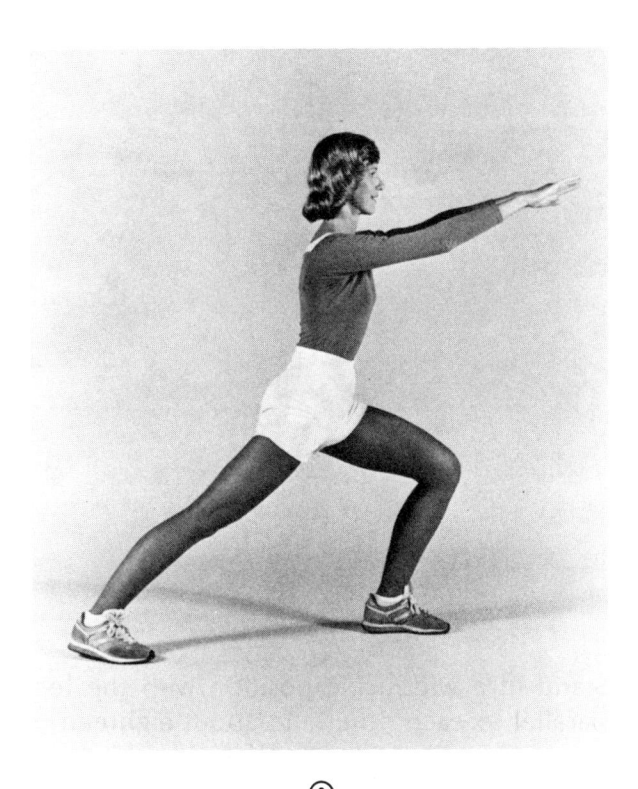

②
Bend the front knee as much as possible while keeping the heels of both feet flat against the floor. Keep the body in a straight plane as much as possible by keeping the buttocks tucked in and the abdomen pulled up and in with the chest lifted and shoulders back. Hold.

③
Repeat ② with the opposite leg in front this time. Hold.

10
Side Lunge

(Legs and buttocks)

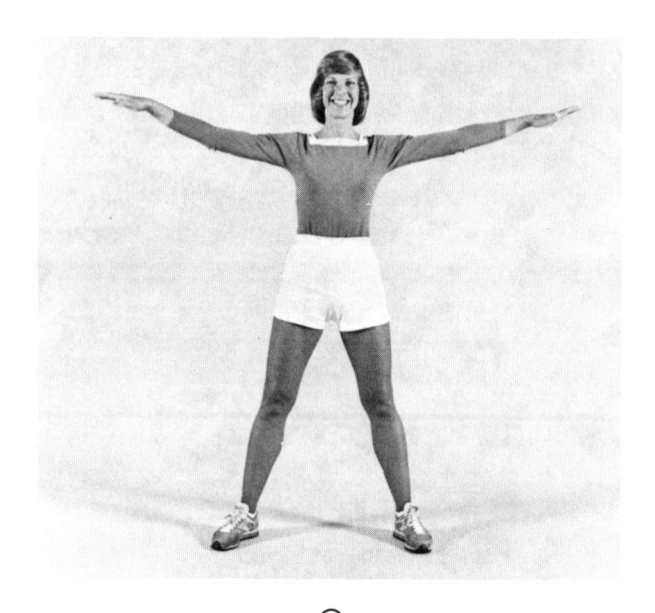

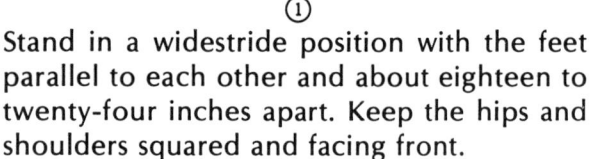

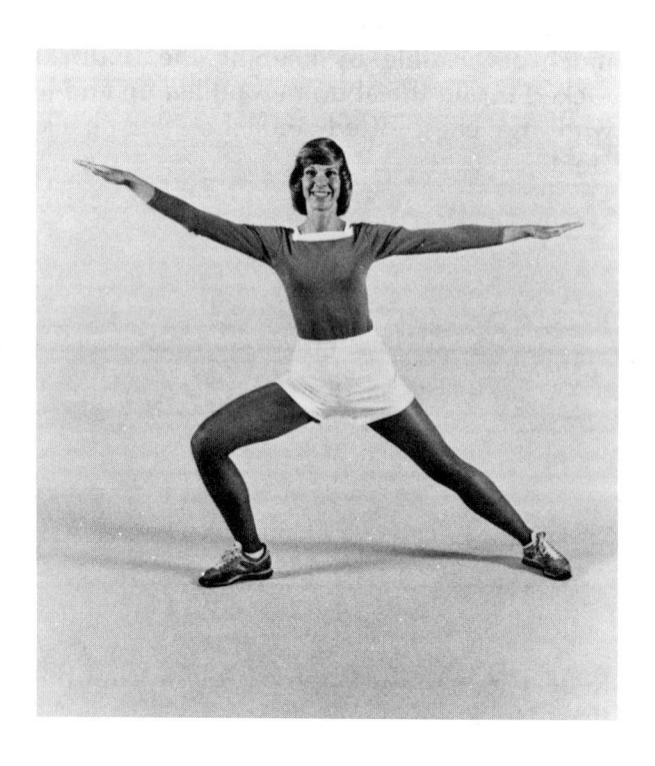

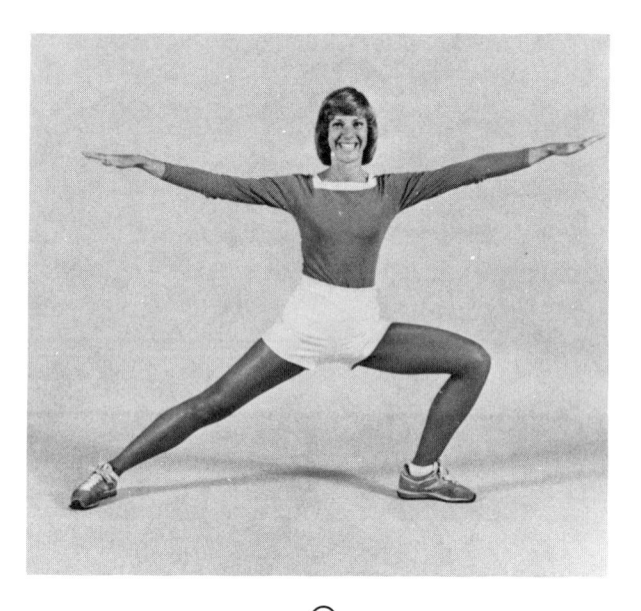

①
Stand in a widestride position with the feet parallel to each other and about eighteen to twenty-four inches apart. Keep the hips and shoulders squared and facing front.

②
Bend one knee to the side as much as possible, keeping both feet flat against the floor. Keep good body alignment with shoulders back, abdomen pulled up and in, rib cage lifted, and buttocks pressed under. Keep the opposite leg straight. Arms are extended outward at shoulder height to help balance. Hold.

③
Repeat ②, bending the opposite knee. Hold.

WARM-UPS: EXERCISES AND ROUTINES 41

11
Big Arm Circles

(Arms and shoulders)

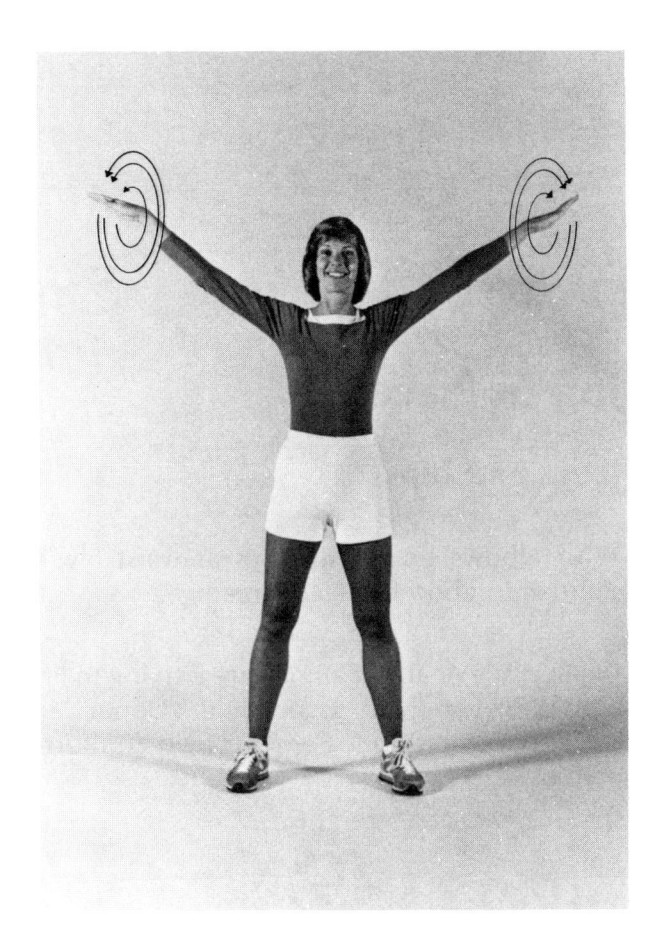

①
Stand with feet comfortably apart with good body alignment. Stretch tall. Extend arms out to side at shoulder height. Keep the elbows straight.

②
Circle arms slowly, making big circles **backward.**

12
Small Arm Circles

(Arms and shoulders)

①
Stand with feet comfortably apart with good body alignment. Stretch tall. Extend the arms out to the side at shoulder level. Keep the elbows straight.

②
Circle arms fast, making small circles as the arms are rotated backward.

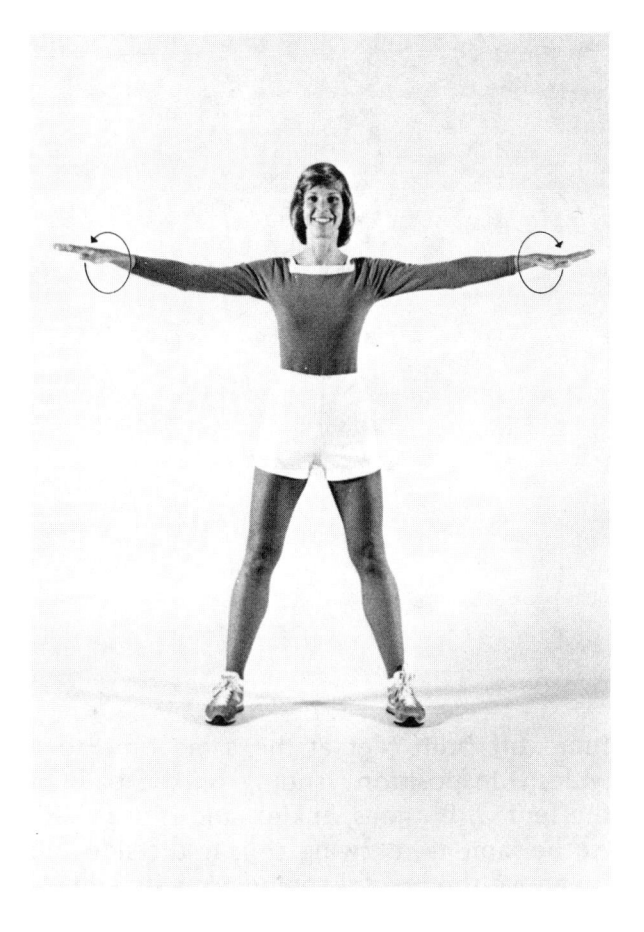

WARM-UPS: EXERCISES AND ROUTINES

13
Jumping Jacks

(Arms, shoulders, and legs)

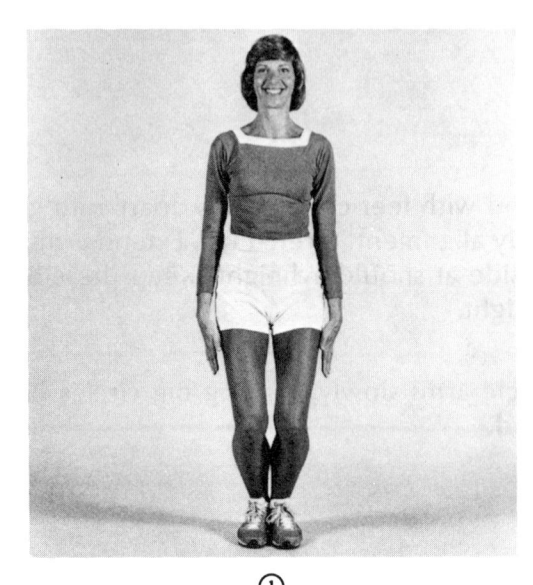

① Stand with feet together, arms at your side, and knees flexed.

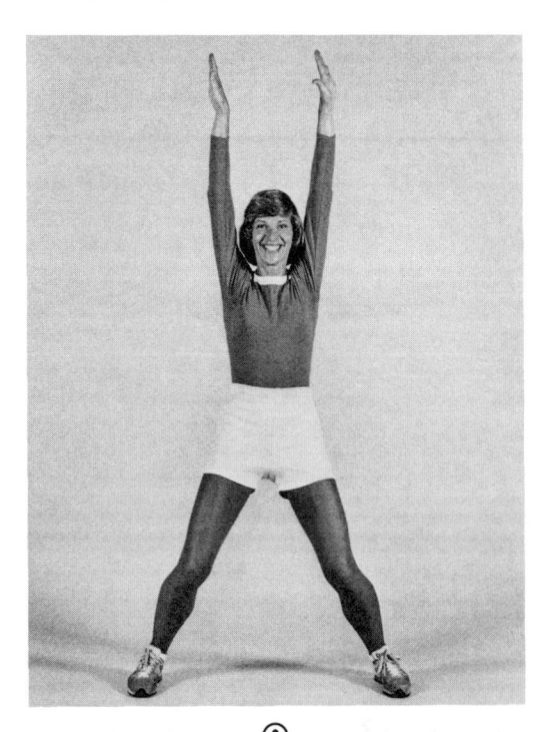

② Jump off both feet at the same time to a widestride position, landing on the balls of the feet with knees, ankles, and hips flexed. At the same time, swing arms to the side and up above the head, keeping arms straight.

③ Jump off both feet and land on the balls of the feet as in position ① with ankles, knees, and hips flexed to absorb the force. Bring arms down to the side. Start comfortably at a rhythmical and slow tempo.

14
Jog In Place

(Legs and hips)

① With elbows bent and arms at waist level, stand with good body alignment.

② Jog in place or about a small area, trying to lift your knees as high as possible. (Upper leg parallel to the floor.) Set your own comfortable pace.

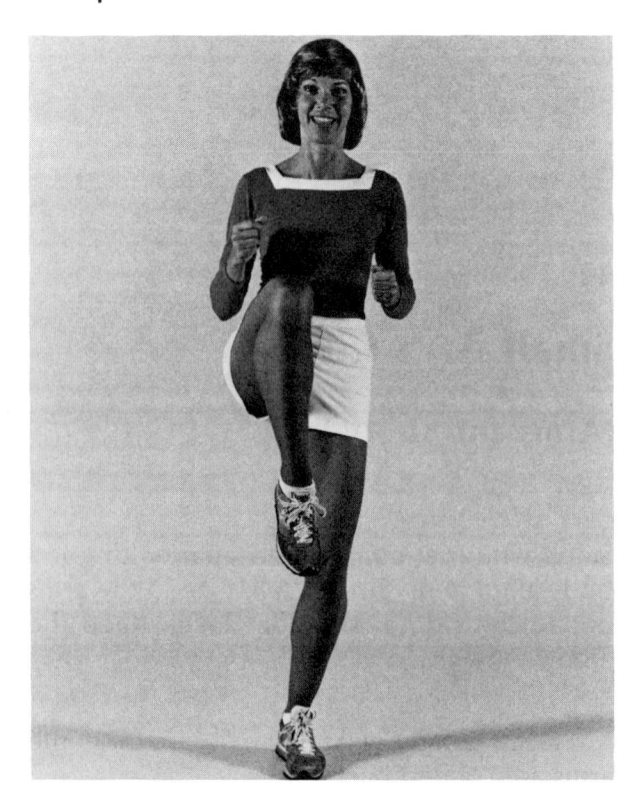

WARM-UP ROUTINE

Music Suggestions (moderate tempo):

- "Elvira," Oak Ridge Boys
- "Sweet Inspiration/Where You Lead," Barbara Streisand
- "Woman In Love," Barbara Streisand
- "Urgent," Foreigner

Exercise	Repetitions	Counts
1 **Head Roll**	4 starting to the right	8 counts each
2 **Shoulder Shrug**	8	4 counts each
3 **Widestride Press** To the right side sit tall To the center sit tall To the left side sit tall To the center sit tall	2 sets	2 counts each movement 16 counts a set
4 **Legs In Front Press**	4	4 counts each movement
5 **Widestride Hug** Press right sit tall Press left sit tall	4 sets	2 counts each movement 8 counts a set
Move from sitting to standing position		8 counts
6 **Lateral Bend** Bend to the right stand tall Bend to the left stand tall	4 sets	2 counts each movement 8 counts a set

WARM-UPS: EXERCISES AND ROUTINES

Exercise	Repetitions	Counts
7		
Front Toe Touch		2 counts each movement
		4 counts a set
Touch down	4 sets	
stretch tall		
8		
Knee Lift		2 counts each movement
		8 counts a set
Lift right knee		
stand tall	4 sets	
Lift left knee		
stand tall		
9		
Twisting Toe Touch		4 counts each movement
To the right	4 sets	8 counts a set
To the left		
10 & 11		
Front and Side Lunges		8 counts each movement
		32 counts a set
Right front		
Left front		
Right side	2 sets	
Left side		
12 & 13		
Big Arm Circles	8	2 counts each
Small Arm Circles	16	1 count each
14		
Jumping Jacks	8	2 counts each
15		
Jog	32	1 count each

SUMMARY

These stretching and flexibility exercises will help loosen and make more supple and flexible the major muscle groups. Start with three to five repetitions and increase the number of repetitions as your physical condition improves. When the exercise says to "hold," do so for approximately two to five seconds. Recover for the same amount of time. Do all exercises at a pace that's comfortable. This will help develop an awareness of which muscles are working and how much improvement is taking place each workout.

5

PERFORMING AEROBIC DANCE ROUTINES

The aerobic dance phase of the workout is a series of gesture and step patterns put to music and performed in a continuous, rhythmical way. Once the dance phase of the program is begun, stay on your feet and keep moving through all aspects of the workout (dancing, walking, pulse taking, etc.). The workout should continue for a minimum of twenty minutes in order to exercise the heart muscle enough to reach your goal of achieving the training effect (pp. 11-12). (**Note:** It may take several workouts of shorter duration for you to become conditioned enough to reach the twenty-minute minimum.)

PACING YOURSELF

Learning to pace yourself during the workout is imperative for you to reach and stay within your training zone. It may be necessary in the beginning to "walk through" (doing the steps without bounce or tension) the dances and then gradually increase the intensity. As you learn and practice the dances, your body will become conditioned to the point where you will be able to bounce more, use greater amounts of tension, lift the knees higher, and get more height in your kicks with less effort.

Pacing can be disrupted by gesture and step patterns that you find difficult. To alleviate this situation, change the difficult gesture and/or step patterns to movements that are easier.

LEARNING THE ROUTINES

Learn one dance at a time. When a dance is mastered, learn a second dance, etc.

Suggestions to help you learn routines are:

①
Learn the step patterns involved in a dance.

②
Count out the beats as you do the routine without music.

③

Concentrate on the transition from one step pattern to the next.

④

Start by walking through the dance slowly, then increase the tempo.

⑤

Familiarize yourself with the music.

⑥

Once you are familiar with the dance, walk through the dance as the music plays.

⑦

Practice the dance to the music using tension, bounce, and an increased heart rate intensity.

⑧

When you feel comfortable putting the step patterns to the music, add the gestures. (Always keep arms at or above waist level.)

Try to keep frustration at a minimum and remember that this isn't a performance — perfection is not necessary. It's only important that you **keep moving** and that you enjoy yourself. Be patient and keep practicing. It becomes easier each time you do a dance.

SELECTING THE MUSIC

Using music that you enjoy — be it rock, jazz, classical, or country and western — adds variety and helps you maintain interest. If you are participating in an aerobic dance class, you may want to substitute songs of your own preference when working out at home on your own.

WHAT IS "A COUNT"?

Listen to your clock — there is a steady beat. Feel your heartbeat — there is a steady beat. Music has a steady beat that is called a count. A beat or count is the unit that measures time. The steady count is the underlying beat to the melody or song.

JAZZ HANDS

You will note that the fingers are spread in many of the pictures. This gesture, called **jazz hands,** helps you tighten the arm and hand muscles, keeping the tension throughout the upper part of the body, not just the legs and feet.

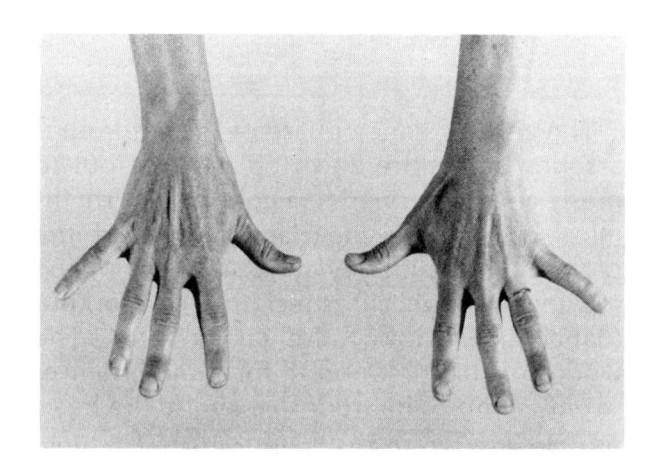

6

COOL DOWNS: EXERCISES AND ROUTINE

PURPOSE OF THE COOL-DOWN PHASE

The cool-down is a term describing the continuation of exercise at a low intensity for a few minutes following a normal workout. Its purpose is to help prevent muscle stiffness and to give your body the opportunity to readjust to the resting or pre-activity state. Cool-down exercises help to speed recovery by removing accumulated metabolic wastes (lactic acid) more rapidly. Abrupt stopping of the dance program may cause stress to the body. The blood could "pool" in the working body parts and cause light-headedness, chills, and/or fainting. Tapering off allows your muscles to help send the extra blood from the extremities back to the heart and brain.

HOW MUCH TIME?

The cool-down phase of the aerobic dance program is as important as the warm-up phase. "A minimum time of five minutes cooling down will give the body the opportunity to recover from the stress of exercise." Continue cooling down until profuse sweating has been curtailed and/or the heart rate is below 120 beats a minute.

WAYS TO COOL DOWN

You can cool down by slowing any large muscle activity. For example, you can "walk" through dance routines or learn an easy, slow-tempoed dance. Walking or jogging slowly for a minimum of five minutes is a good transition between aerobic activity and resting.

In other words, you need to cool down the body the same way that you warm up by a gradual change in the tempo of the activity. This can be accomplished by gradually diminishing your intensity level. This can also be accomplished by using stretching exercises after the aerobic dance workout. Note that after the cool-down phase of the total workout, relaxation and breathing exercises are added to help the body cool down. (Suggestion: after working out, a lukewarm shower or bath will also promote relaxation.)

A Reminder: The exercises used for warm-ups can also be used for cool-downs by just reversing the order. You begin from a slow walking, to a sitting, and finally to a lying down position for the cool-down.

COOL-DOWN EXERCISES

1
Tailor Sitting, Straight Back Press
(Inner thighs and back)

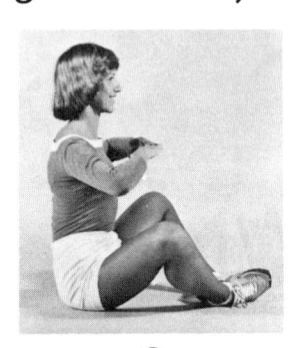

①
Sit with soles of feet together, knees pointing sideward. Pull feet as close to the body as possible. Bend elbows and place arms at shoulder level. Pull spine straight and shoulders back. Pull shoulder blades as close together as possible. Hold this back position for the entire exercise.

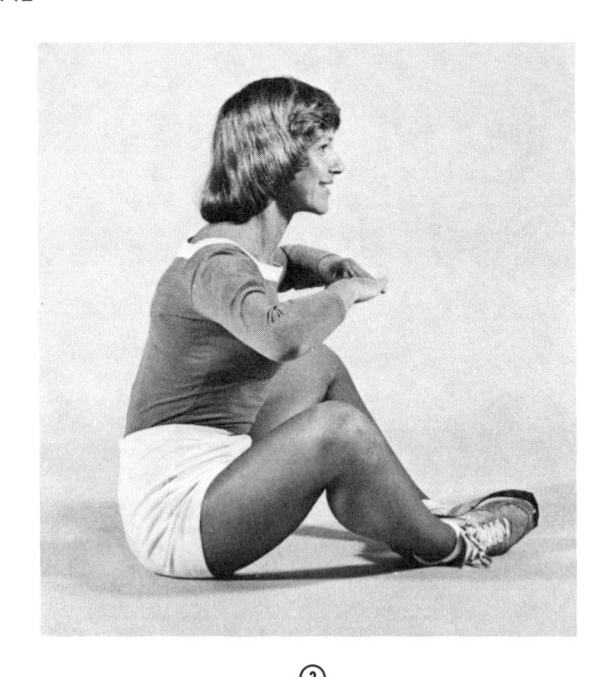

②
Slowly press forward from the hips as far as possible, keeping the back straight and the head in alignment with the back. Hold.

③
Return to starting position ①. Hold.

2
Widestride Sitting, Straight Back Press
(Back and legs)

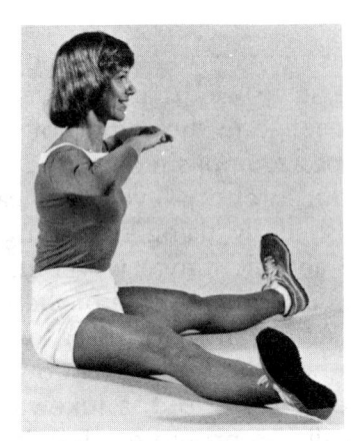

①
Sit with legs straight and as far apart as is comfortable in the widestride position. The knees and toes are pointed upward, the heels pressed forward. The arms are straight and extended upward above the head.

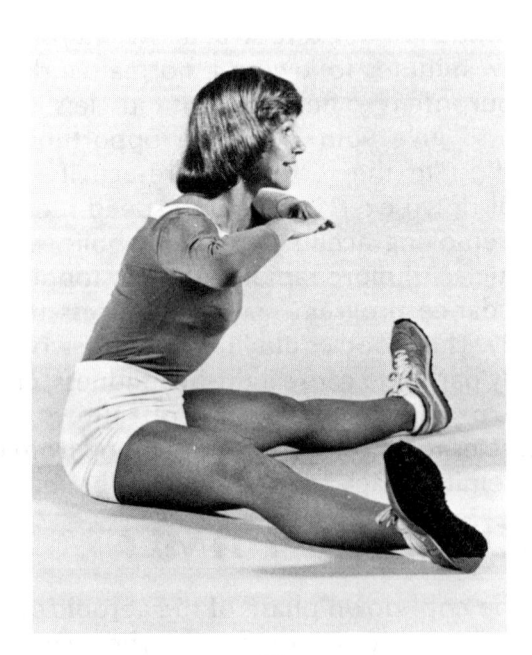

②
Slowly press forward from the hips as far as possible, keeping the back straight and the head in alignment with the back. Hold.

③
Return to position ①. Hold.

COOL DOWNS: EXERCISES AND ROUTINE 49

3
Widestride Sitting, Rounded Back Press
(Back and legs)

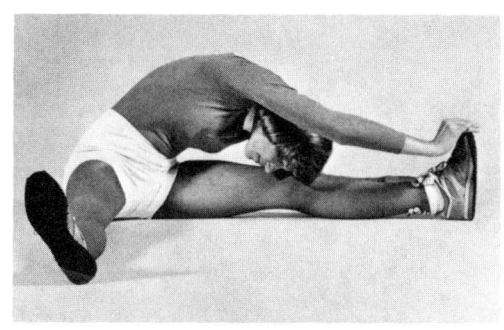

① Sit with legs straight and comfortably apart. The knees and toes are pointed upward with the heels pressed forward. The arms are straight and are extended upward above the head.

② Stretch the arms and bend with rounded back toward the left knee with the nose leading. Press and hold.

③ Return to position ①. Hold.

4
Straight Legs, Straight Back Press
(Legs and back)

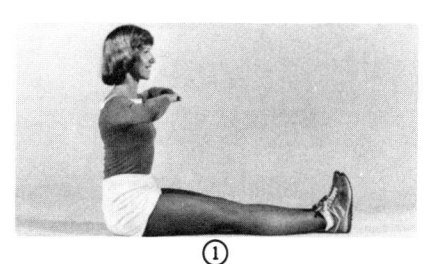

① Sit with legs straight and together in front of you. The knees and toes are pointed upward; the heels are pressed forward. The back is straight with the shoulders back, arms at shoulder level, and elbows bent.

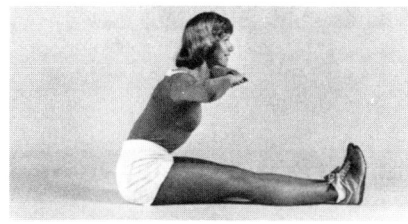

② Slowly press forward from the hips as far as possible, keeping the back straight with the head in alignment with the back. Hold.

③ Return to position ①. Hold.

5
Knee to Chest Pull

(Lower back and hips)

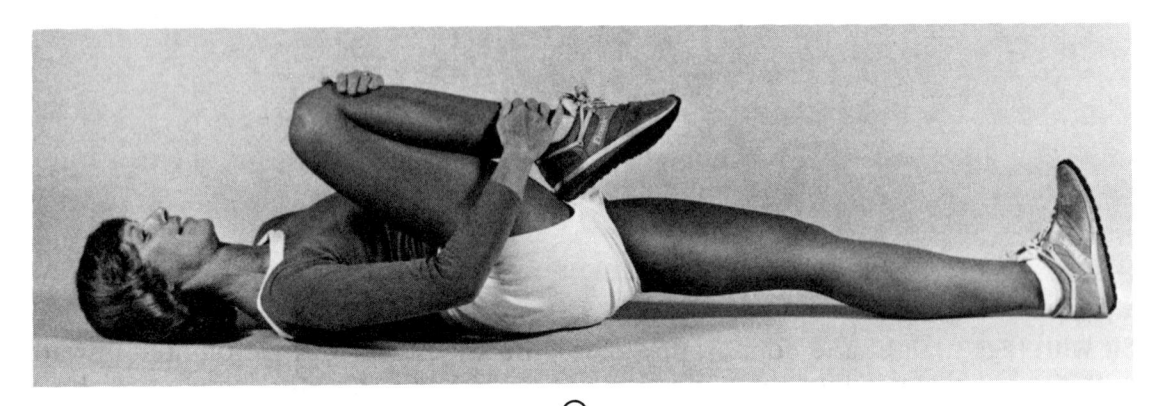

① Lie on your back with both legs extended, together and straight.

② Grasp the right leg below the knee as you bend the right knee slowly, pulling it tightly against your chest. Hold, keeping the other leg flat on the floor.

③ Repeat ② with the left knee.

④ Return to ① position.

6
Both Knees to Chest Pull

(Lower back and hips)

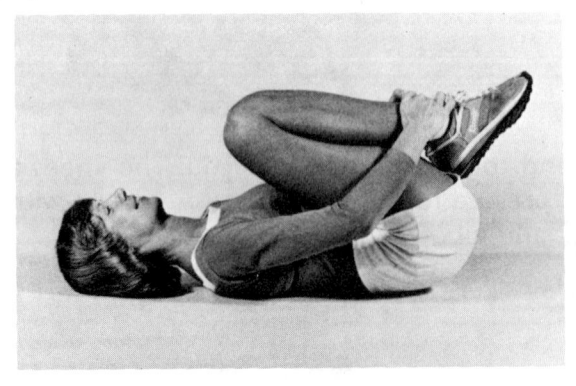

① Lying on your back, extend both legs so that they are straight and together.

② Grasp the legs below the knees as you bend both knees slowly toward your chest. Pull the knees tightly against your chest. Hold.

③ Return to ① position by keeping the knees bent and then sliding feet out once they are touching the floor, straightening the legs.

COOL DOWNS: EXERCISES AND ROUTINE 51

7
Leg Extension Press
(Legs and back)

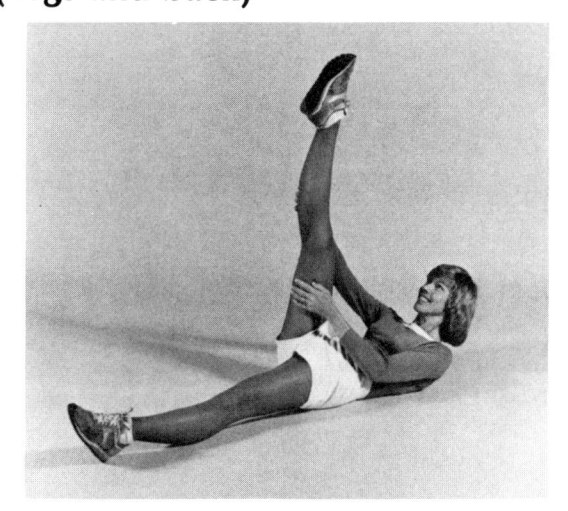

①
Lying on your back, extend both legs until they are straight and together on the floor.
②
Bend the right knee to your chest, and extend the leg upward until it is straight and perpendicular with the floor; head may be raised or on the floor.

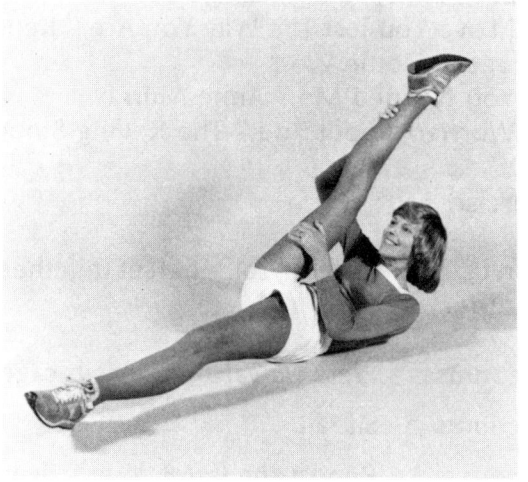

③
Return to ① position.
④
Repeat ②, bending the left knee to your chest, then extending the left leg. Hold.
⑤
Return to ① position.

8
Total Body Stretch
(Entire body)

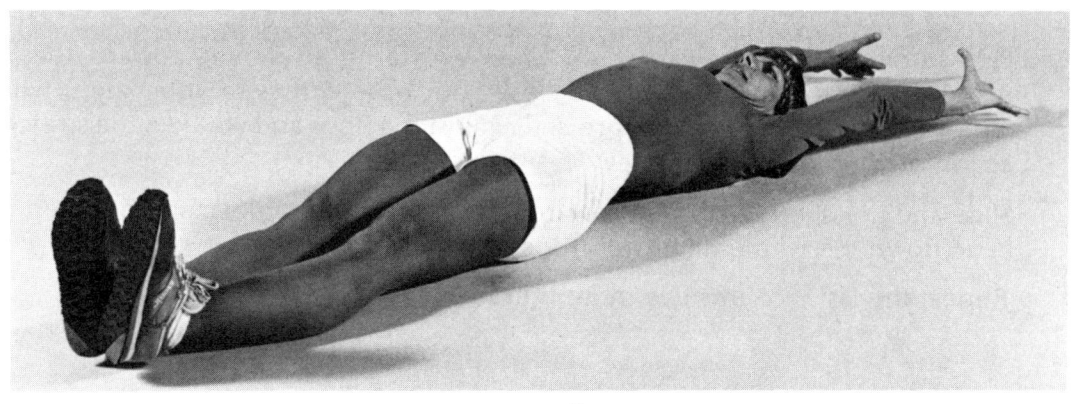

①
Lie on your back with arms and legs against the floor. The arms are straight, reaching above the head. The legs are straight down from your hips and are placed together.
②
Point and widely stretch fingers and flex ankles forward, heels pressing as you tense every muscle in your body, and stretch as far as you comfortably can. Hold.
③
Relax all the muscles, feeling the tension lessen throughout the entire body.

COOL-DOWN ROUTINE

Suggested Music:

- "Even Now," Barry Manilow
- "I Love You Just The Way You Are," Kenny Rogers, Dottie West
- "You Needed Me," Anne Murray
- "Worried About You," The Rolling Stones

Exercise 1

Sit in tailor-sit fashion, soles of feet together, elbows bent, back straight the whole time, head up, not forward.

4 counts	Press forward (lifting rib cage as you press).
4 counts	Sit tall.
40 counts	Repeat the last 8 counts **five** more times.

Exercise 2

Sit in a widestride position, press heels forward, with elbows bent, back straight (no rounded shoulders), head held up, chin level.

4 counts	Press forward (lifting rib cage as you press).
4 counts	Sit tall.
40 counts	Repeat the last 8 counts **five** more times.

Exercise 3

Sit in a widestride sitting position, press heels forward, keep legs flat on floor.

4 counts	Press, bringing nose toward right knee with arms stretching toward toes (remember — it doesn't matter how close your nose comes to your knee; what is important is that your legs stay pressed against the floor and you feel the stretching action of your working muscles).
4 counts	Slide and press, bringing nose toward left knee for the same exercise. (Keep your head down the whole time; no sitting up at all.)
40 counts	Repeat the last 8 counts **five** more times.

Exercise 4

Sit with legs together and straight in front of you, elbows bent, back straight, head in alignment with your spine.

4 counts	Press forward (lifting rib cage as you do).
4 counts	Sit tall.
40 counts	Repeat the last 8 counts **five** more times.

Exercise 5

Lie on your back, with left leg stretched against the floor straight down from the hip and the right knee pulled to your chest with your hands, keeping calf against thigh the whole time. (Head can be against floor or curled toward chest.)

4 counts	Pull your right knee tight against your chest.
4 counts	Relax, keeping right knee near your chest.
40 counts	Repeat the last 8 counts **five** more times.
4 counts	Pull your left knee tight against your chest.
4 counts	Relax, keeping left knee near your chest.
40 counts	Repeat last 8 counts **five** more times.

Exercise 6

4 counts	Pull both knees tight against your chest.
4 counts	Relax, keeping both knees near your chest.
40 counts	Repeat the last 8 counts **five** more times.

Exercise 7

Continue lying on your back (with head curled or resting against the floor), keep the left leg extended against the floor straight down from your hip, toe and ankle flexed, and lift the right leg so that it is perpendicular to the floor. Press right leg back toward your head. Your shoulders and arms are on the floor.

4 counts	Press leg toward your head.
4 counts	Relax leg in starting position.
40 counts	Repeat last 8 counts **five** more times.
4 counts	Press left leg toward your head.
4 counts	Relax leg in starting position.
40 counts	Repeat last 8 counts **five** more times.

Exercise 8

Lower your leg and place arms along the floor above the head.

8 counts	Stretch the total body as far as you comfortably can, tensing every muscle in your body.
8 counts	Relax the muscles, taking as much tension out of the body as possible.

STRENGTH DEVELOPMENT

If you are interested in incorporating a strength program, **now** is the time in your workout program to do so. You do strength activities to "thicken those rubber bands" you have as muscles, and you allow them to endure longer periods of work **after** an aerobic workout so that you do not begin aerobics in oxygen-debt (fatigued or out-of-breath).

The two most popular strength activities that can be used easily in an aerobic dance setting are push-ups and bent-knee sit-ups. Positions for the beginner and more advanced are both presented here.

9
Modified Push-Up
(Arms, shoulders, and chest)

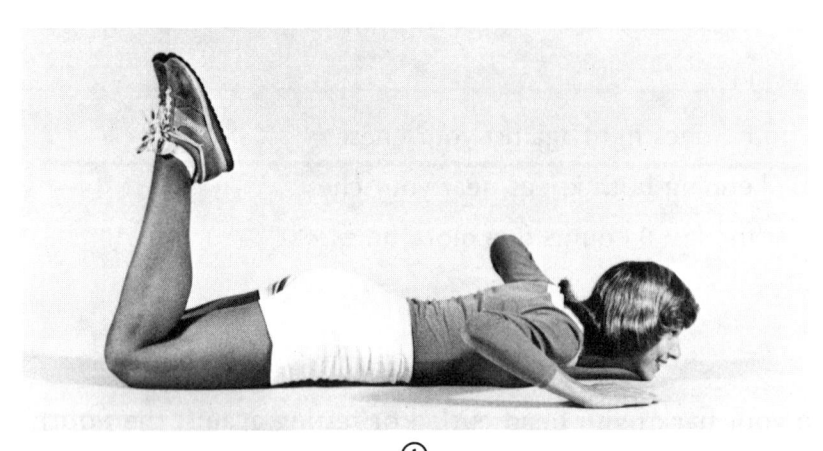

①
Lie in a prone position on the floor. Place hands under your shoulders, fingers forward. Feet are together, pointing upward, with the knees together and bearing the weight. Inhale before Step ②.

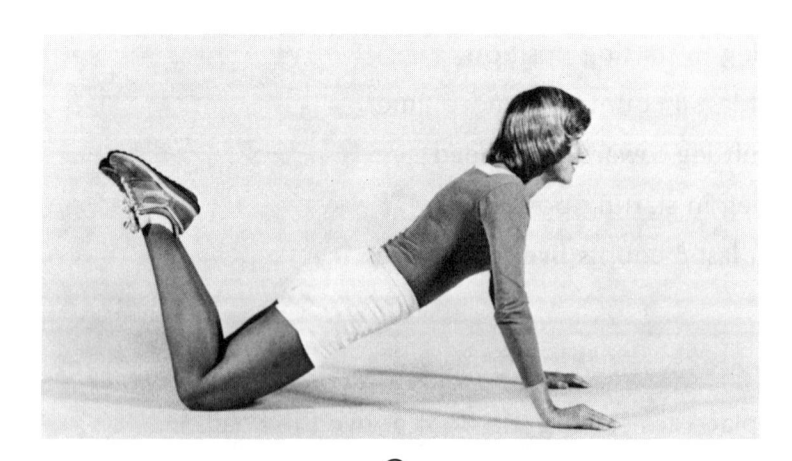

②
Keep the body a **straight** plane from the knees to the head as you push the upper part of your body off the floor until your arms are completely extended. Exhale as you do this step.

③
Lower your body until nose touches the floor, inhaling as you recover. Begin with one push-up and gradually increase the repetitions until you are able to do twenty. Remember to rhythmically breathe. **Don't** hold your breath.

COOL DOWNS: EXERCISES AND ROUTINE 55

10
Push-Up
(Arms, shoulders, and chest)

①
Lie in a prone position on the floor. Place hands under your shoulders, fingers forward and feet together, taking weight on the **balls** of the feet. Inhale before Step ②.

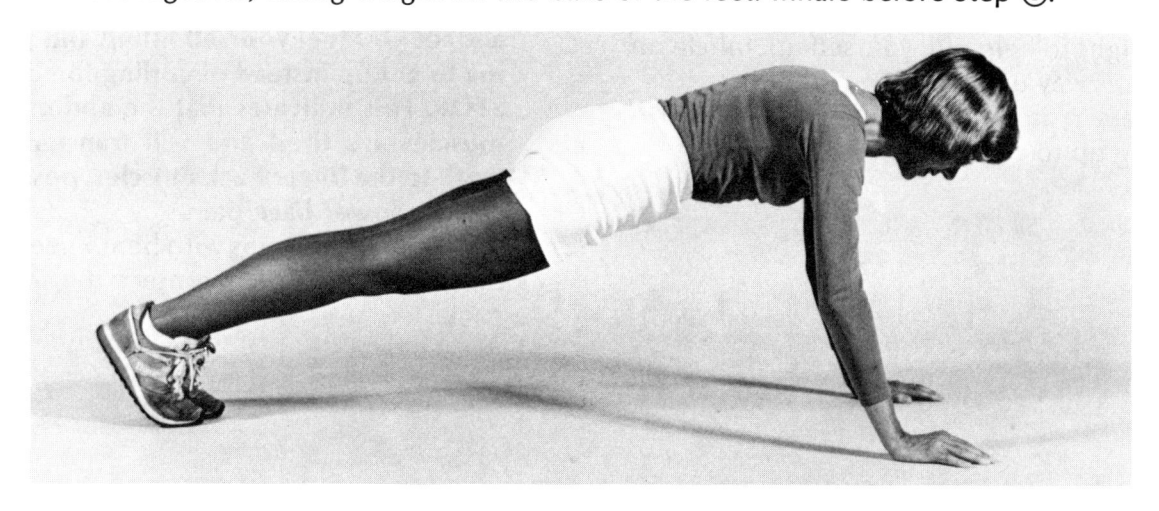

②
Keep the body straight as you push up until both arms are straight. Exhale as you do this step.

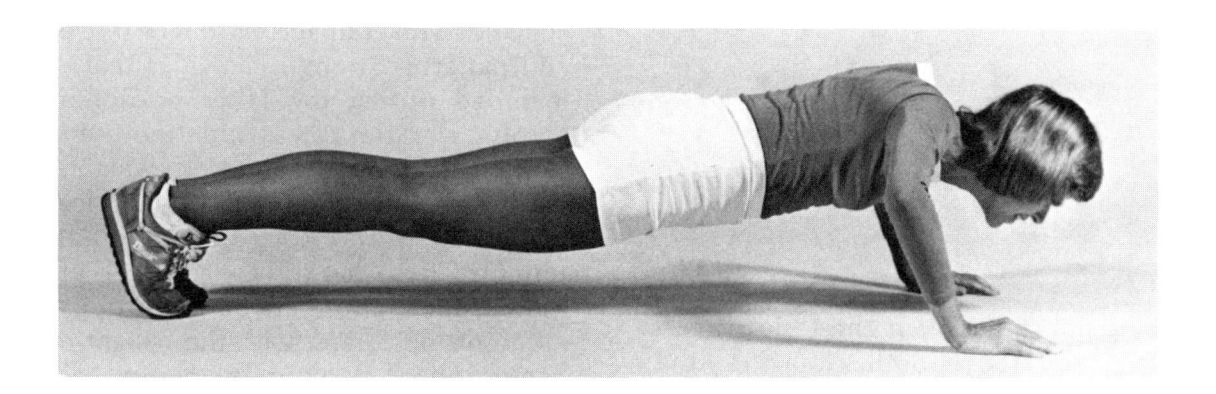

③
Lower your body halfway to the floor by bending your elbows, keeping the weight equally distributed on your hands and the balls of your feet.

Begin with one push-up and gradually increase the repetitions until you are doing twenty. It will take several weeks to reach this goal. Remember to keep the head straight. Pulling the head upward may cause the lower back to sag and could be harmful.

Note: Keep the lower back from arching. Also, do not raise buttocks to dip chin.

11
Bent-Knee Sit-Up
(Abdomen)

To begin conditioning:
- Use your hands and arms to help you sit up if you cannot do the following exercise without using them. Lie with arms at your side. Put your hands under your thighs to help pull yourself up. Inhale on your way up.
- Repeat as many times as you can, working up to twenty.

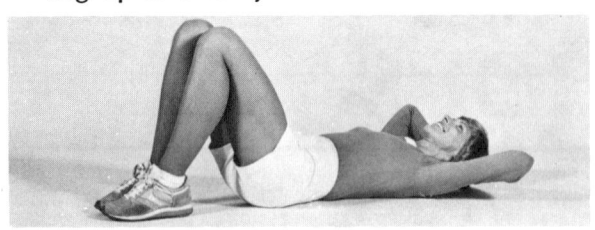

①

For advanced persons:
Lie on your back with hands clasped behind the head. Bend knees skyward and bring your feet, flat on the floor, about one foot from your buttocks.

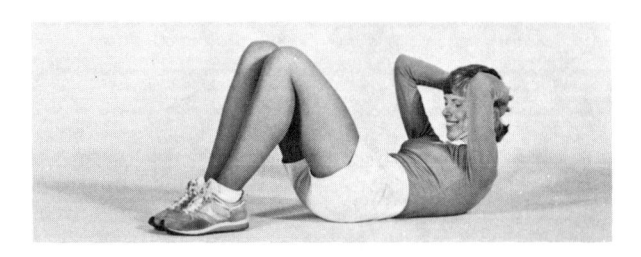

②

Tucking the chin to your chest, slowly **curl** forward and touch both elbows to the knees. Inhale on your way up.

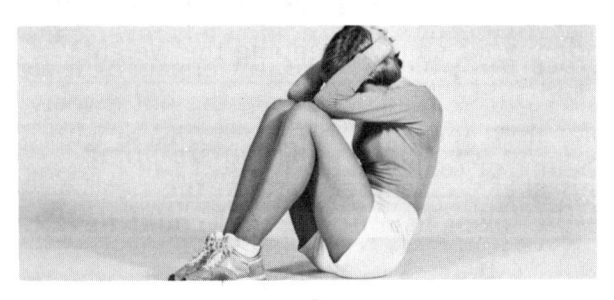

③

Return to ① position by curling backward, keeping chin tucked and back rounded. Exhale on your way down.

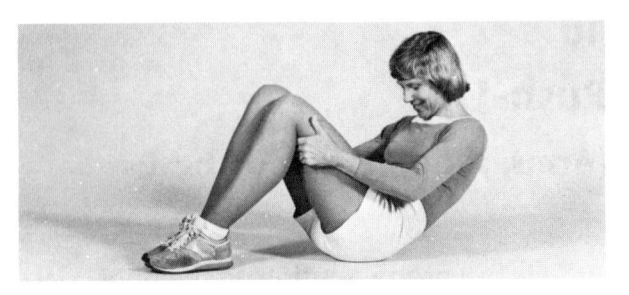

- **CAUTION: If the muscles start to quiver and/or you feel yourself lifting and jerking to get up instead of curling the back, STOP. This indicates that the abdominal muscles are tired and will transfer the work to the lower back muscles, possibly causing lower back pain.**
- Always do the sit-ups with bent knees for the same reason: to protect the lower back.

ADD VARIETY

Also, after you become cardiorespiratory fit, try a little variety by incorporating strength activities **with** your aerobic dance movements and patterns. Strength activities that can be included during the **latter** portion of the aerobic workout can include the use of free weights held in your hands, or weights worn around the ankles. (Homemade sandbags are inexpensive.) The development of strength **requires,** then, that you progressively increase the weight(s) and that you go through a full range of movement with the weight in your hands and/or on your ankles. So, you must continually stress stretching the muscles and flexing in each direction the associated joints will go — to joint extreme — not just having them "in place" and **hanging** there.

Briefly now, cool-down again and follow with the relaxation presented next.

7
VOLUNTARY CONSCIOUS RELAXATION

*"When you can get in touch
With an inner quietness —
A mental pool of renewed energy —
Who then can possibly enter?"*

Developing **total control** of your mind and body is an awesome goal and one for which we all strive, consciously or unconsciously. It seems to take the gift of supreme self-discipline, with which few of us are intuitively blessed, to master total control with ease. Most of us must therefore "work at it" by educating our bodies and minds first. Only through the repetitious practice of the skill we wish to master will we obtain the self-discipline. This is true for attaining either total physical control or total mental control. **Repetition and practice** are the keys to the total control for which we strive.

Developing total control of our minds to allow us to master relaxation sounds like a uniquely powerful skill. And it can be — **if** each individual allows himself or herself the time to learn and practice this skill. For total relaxation **is** a skill that must be mastered. A few individuals may be able to totally relax without any training — but we've yet to meet even one.

YOU'VE EARNED IT — LET'S RELAX

Have you ever enjoyed an exercise session and left all hot, sweaty, and tired — but happy, just knowing you've done something positive for yourself? Have you, likewise, ever thought how terrific it would be to leave just happy (minus the hot, sweaty, and tired feeling)? If so, you've probably never realized there is another step, or routine procedure, that you need to do to completely reverse the process in which you've just engaged! It allows you to totally eliminate the hot, sweaty, and tired feelings. You instead leave with a feeling of renewed energy (we call it being "energized"). (All this and no shower yet!)

Very simply, here is what happens to your body following sustained, **strenuous** (not light) exercise, like the aerobic dance you have just engaged in for twenty to sixty minutes:

①

Beta endorphins, which are natural brain hormones (neuropeptides) with effects similar to those of morphine, and which play a major (but not total) role in the body's control of pain,[1] are released. These hormones then travel from the brain to the spinal fluid, and subsequently to all nervous tissue. (Again, this has been found to occur **only** during sustained physical exertion — not during just any light exercise session.)

②

All body nervous tissues receive these natural hormone drugs that have been produced and released, and a glow envelopes you. The feeling is described as a "natural high."

③

Your heart rate following the cool-down exercises/routine will lower to approximately the rate taken during the warm-up stretching portion of the hour, and breathing will be easier.

④

Most of the sweating mechanism will begin to subside.

It is now time to incorporate three to fifteen minutes of total relaxation into your fitness program. During this time, the tension previously held in all muscle groups is eliminated as much as possible. You can master this goal **with practice** in the minimum amount of time of approximately two or three minutes.[2] The training period to allow you to master the technique of relaxation will take about five or ten minutes at the conclusion of each aerobic dance session for approximately ten weeks. (When relaxation is practiced before going to bed, or during the middle of the day, fifteen minutes of practice is suggested.) We have found it easier for beginners to attempt relaxation through practice **after** a sustained exercise session, rather than during or after various daily activities.[3]

You will usually find at the conclusion of this technique that:

①

Your sweating mechanism will have completely stopped.

②

Your breathing rate and body temperature will be back to your normal range.

③

Your heart rate will most likely be lower than when you arrived, and for many will even be approaching (or at) your resting heart rate![4]

All of this with only three minutes of effort following the cool-down!

VOLUNTARY CONSCIOUS RELAXATION

This technique differs greatly from many other equally effective methods. It totally uses your powers of control through your **imagination** — your mind seeks out and recognizes tension. It then eliminates it, again through your ability to imagine the relaxation. No physical exertion or planned tensing of muscle groups is performed.

There are four steps to voluntary conscious relaxation:

①

Establishing the relaxation position.

②

Establishing the breathing pattern.

③

"Tuning-in" to various parts of the body.

④

Heart rate monitoring followed by simple static stretching to make each person alert again (unless the technique is used prior to going to bed).

STEP I — ESTABLISHING THE RELAXATION POSITION

①

Lie on your back. If you feel uncomfortable because your entire back is not in contact with the floor, raise one knee up with your foot flat on the floor, approximately one foot from your buttocks. (Persons with either substantial buttocks or shoulder mass will find that this "knee up" position will relieve the arched lower back feeling.)

②

Turn your head slightly to one side. When you become totally relaxed, your tongue will relax backward and cover your windpipe if you keep your head straight in line with the rest of you.

③

Place your arms on the floor at your sides, palms down, with elbows a little bent. Flexed joints are more relaxed.

④

Place your legs a bit apart (not crossed or in contact with one another). As the legs relax, your feet will tend to roll outward.

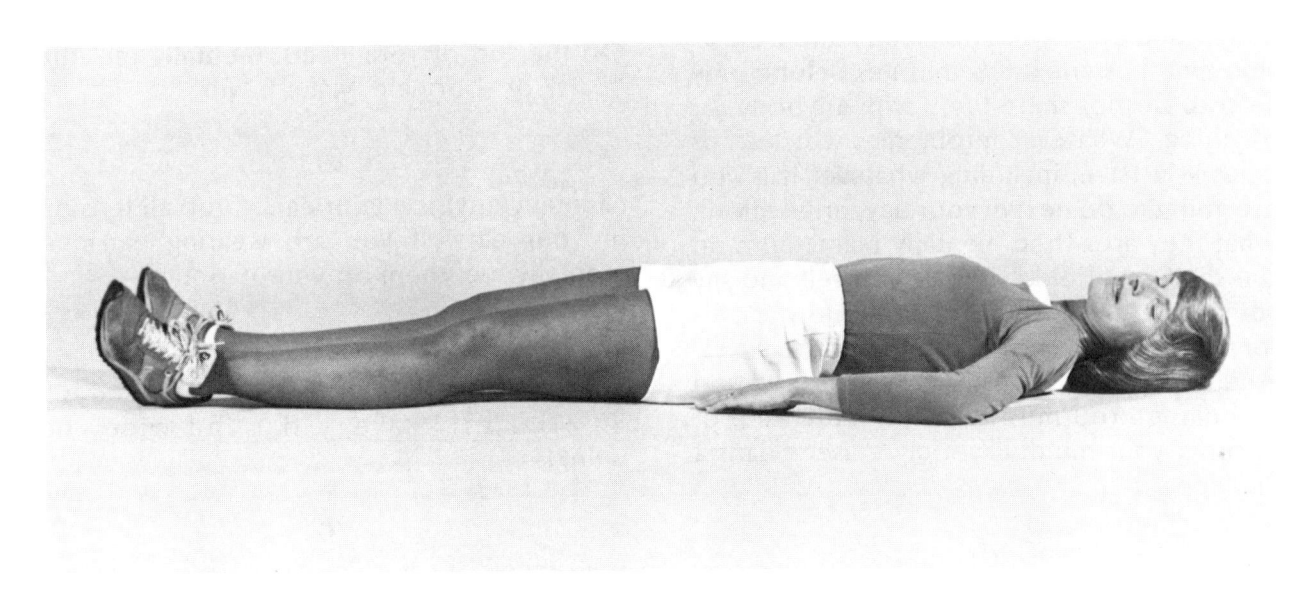

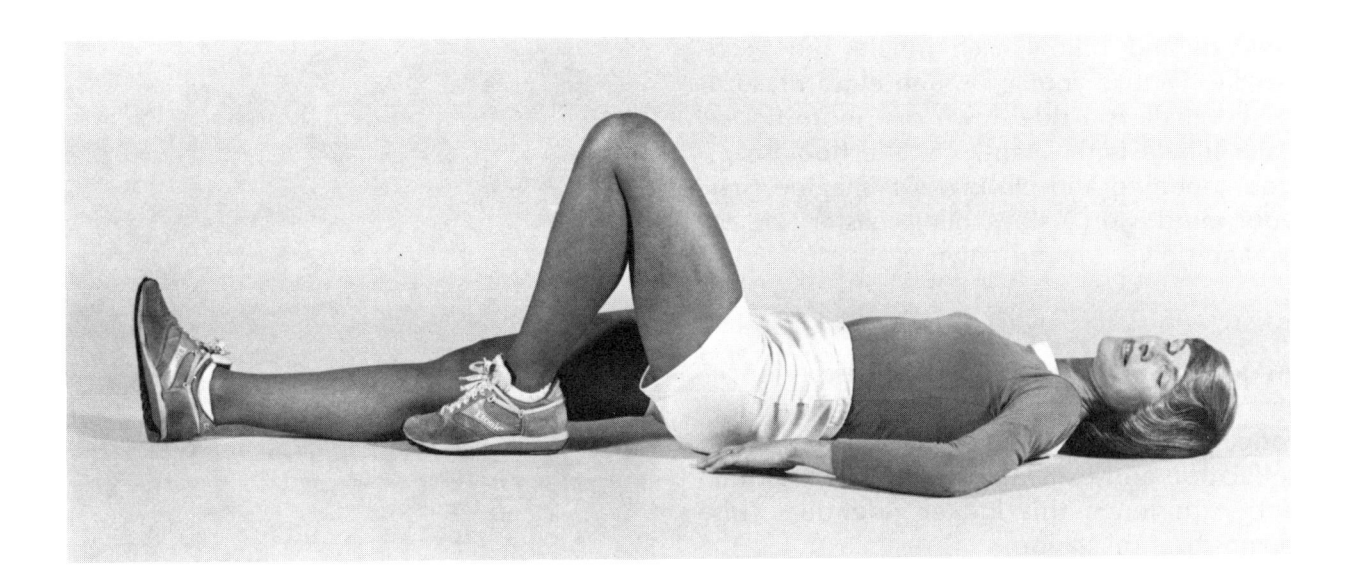

VOLUNTARY CONSCIOUS RELAXATION

⑤

If you consciously relax best with your eyes open, keep them open. If you consciously relax best with your eyes closed, close them. If you keep them open, focus **continually** on **one** object only.

STEP II — ESTABLISHING THE BREATHING PATTERN

①

Take one deep breath and exhale slowly. Determine during this inhalation and exhalation that these next few minutes **belong only to you.** Do not share them with anybody, or anything. Whatever problems, worries, or cares you have, including whatever it is you are going to do next in your day, briefly think what they are. Then mentally place them on the shelf on "hold." Talk to yourself and say something like, "This is my time now (problem) and you are just going to have to wait." And then forget it during your relaxation technique! You must take this initial step of clearing your mind, like a big eraser cleans a chalkboard.

②

Now follow your breathing cycle, whether it is fast, slow, regular, or irregular. Just mentally tune in and follow each inhale and each exhale. Picture yourself on an elevator, and each exhale is a ride down one more floor; each inhale is the pause for the floor stop, door opening and closing. Or imagine that your mind is on a slow roller coaster ride of up and down, up and down.

③

As you begin to relax, you will experience that the exhalation (breathing out) becomes longer and longer. Don't interfere with your inhalation and exhalation — just ride with it and experience this longer ride out. **This begins true relaxation.**

④

At various times during the entire voluntary conscious relaxation technique, you will have to mentally tune back in to your breathing technique, for mastering this "roller coaster ride" is the **central focus** of your total control over relaxation.

STEP III — TUNING IN TO VARIOUS PARTS OF THE BODY

We'll start at the top of your head and travel down to the tips of your toes.

①

On the top of your head, **mentally** feel the "part" of your hair. Make it wide.

②

Mentally envision your ears. Drop all tension in your ears. If you are wearing earrings, mentally feel them on your earlobes.

③

Tune-in to your forehead. Is it tense and full of wrinkles? Make it flat and wide; no wrinkles.

④

What is the space between your eyebrows doing? Is it grooved and full of wrinkles?

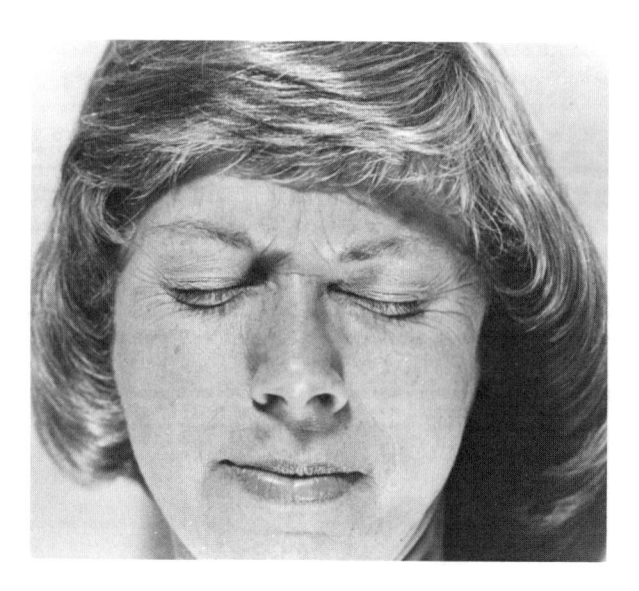

Relax, with a wide space between your eyebrows. This is one of **the** telltale locations of human stress. A person who is highly stressed seems to permanently keep the space between the eyebrows tensed (contracted, wrinkled). Calm, serene people stand out by having this small space wide, relaxed, and untensed.

⑤

Relax your eyebrows as if heavy weights were pulling down the ends. This will also relax your temple area.

⑥

There is a hinge joint near your ear that is used to open and close your lower jaw. Relax that joint by dropping your lower jaw. It will make your lips part. Relax your chin.

⑦

When you relax your jaw, mentally feel your teeth and tongue. When some people try to practice total relaxation, they tightly press (tense) their tongue to the roof of their mouths. Also, many people grit or grind their teeth at night — an audible sign of tension in the area.

⑧

Relax your throat by thinking of the feeling you get with the second stage of swallowing. Persons who sing or play musical instruments have been trained in this technique to relax the area so that the best sounds will come out.

⑨

Drop your shoulders and chest so that there is a wide space between your ears and shoulders. This is an area that we unconsciously tense throughout the day, unnecessarily. Whether we drive a car or walk in miserable weather, we tense the shoulders up near our ears and encourage neck aches and headaches. When you think about it next time, untense this group if you don't actually need to be holding it in a tensed manner.

⑩

Allow the weight of your chest to sink through to the floor. Think: heavy chest.

⑪

Drop all tension from your upper arms, elbows, lower arms, and hands until you can just feel your fingertips pulsating on the floor. A tingling feeling may be felt in your fingertips.

Drop your shoulders and chest so that there is a wide space between your ears and your shoulders.

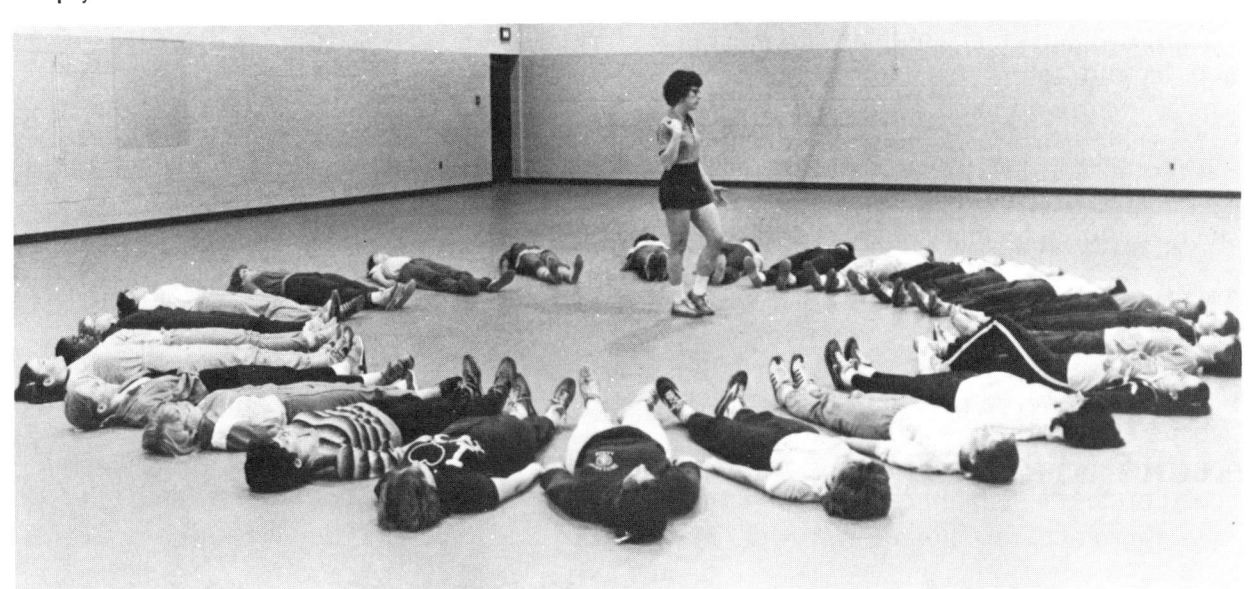

⑫

Relax your kneecaps. This joint connects your upper and lower leg, and many times we tense our knee area when we attempt to relax other body parts. When you relax the knees, the upper legs will relax, and the heavy weight of your legs will begin to drop to the floor. Likewise, the lower legs respond almost automatically, with the feet then rolling outward.

⑬

Mentally feel what your toes are doing in your shoes. Are they tensed and curled under? If so, relax them.

⑭

And now, return to the most difficult place to relax — the stomach and intestinal area. Begin by first relaxing the buttocks. Now turn your mind back to the navel area and picture a wide, flat, picturesque pond. Envision a small pebble being tossed into the very center, with a soft, rippling effect occurring. Each ripple is a wave of relaxation. Feel the weight of your navel area sinking through, past your spine, onto the floor below you.

⑮

Now return back to your breathing cycle and follow it several times.

⑯

And finally, retake a mental check of all body parts, beginning at the top part of your hair, traveling down to your toes, and finishing with your navel area.

⑰

Now just **rest** a few minutes and enjoy the totally untensed feeling you are experiencing.

STEP IV — HEART RATE MONITORING AND ALERT STRETCH

①

In this lying down position, feel for your pulse. Mentally picture and feel your heart beating. Actively try to slow it down with your mind — tell it to go slower.

②

Count your pulse for fifteen seconds and multiply by four for a minute heart rate count. How does this compare with your pre-activity heart rate count and your resting heart rate count? Isn't it phenomenal what three minutes of relaxation can do for your body's recovery from exercise?

③

You can now leave feeling totally renewed, refreshed, and in control of what remains of the rest of the day!

④

Before you get up, **sit up** and slowly stretch your arms, legs, chest, back, etc. so that you become **alert** immediately. You must do this fifteen-second stretch, or you'll find yourself yawning for an hour afterwards! Of course, if this relaxation procedure is practiced before going to bed, omit this "alert stretch."

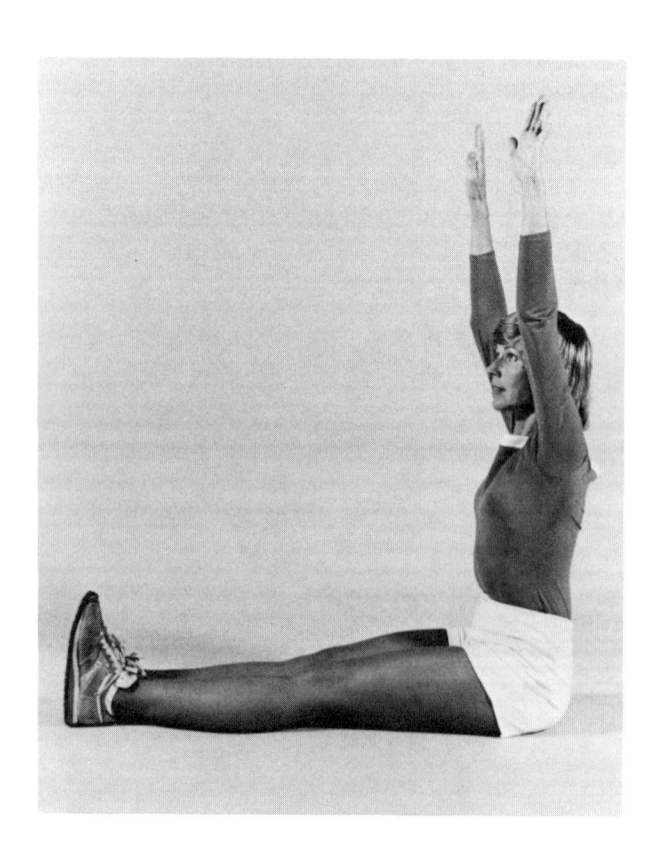

The aforementioned steps were given in the form of mental cueing. Say and do each step **slowly** so that it takes on meaning. Perhaps you can tape your own voice, giving each cue slowly and playing it to yourself as you practice the skill of relaxation at home. It would be a lot easier than reading the cues to yourself and then trying to apply them during the relaxation.

When you have mastered this technique and developed total relaxation for yourself, you will find that you can apply this technique anywhere (with only slight changes in body position, etc.). **You can then incorporate this relaxation technique to all moments of stress** and develop total mental control. When you are in total control of your mind, in all circumstances, **no one** can bug you!

8

CHOREOGRAPHING YOUR OWN ROUTINES

To choreograph your own routines, choose your favorite music with a moderate to fast tempo. Use songs that are upbeat and that give you a good feeling. Make sure that you will enjoy your choices, because you will be hearing them a lot — first as you choreograph and then as you dance. Remember that the dances you have learned and will be choreographing can be performed to different musical selections. Each dance doesn't have to be performed to the same song every time. The music that you select can be your best motivator to keep you dancing aerobically on a regular basis.

GUIDELINES FOR CHOREOGRAPHING

The following guidelines will help you choreograph your own routines:

①
Your dance does not need to last as long as the song.

②
You can choreograph one sequence and keep repeating it until the music is over.

③
You can choreograph two sequences and combine them in any way you want. For example, 1-2-1-2 (as in "Don't Stop Till You Get Enough") or 1-1-2; 1-1-2 (as in "Ride Like The Wind") (see Chapter 5).

④
Make the dance sequencing easy to learn and remember. If it becomes too complicated and you spend a lot of time learning it, you defeat the purpose of doing an aerobic dance — that purpose is to keep moving without stopping.

CHOREOGRAPHING YOUR OWN ROUTINES

(5)

As you create your dances, make sure that you sequence steps so you are moving continuously without any stopping.

(6)

You can pace the routine by putting in steps like the lunge, arm swings, walks, etc. that allow *some* "slowing down" but *not* stopping. This is an especially useful technique for songs like "Copacabana" that last a long time. Of course, a dance of longer duration comes in your program after you've been aerobic dancing for at least six to nine sessions (a minimum of twenty minutes of aerobic dancing each session).

(7)

Keep your arms above your waist at all times. When you are first learning the footwork, you don't need to choreograph the arms yet. You do need to keep them in a jogger's position (explained in Chapter 5) or at least above the waist. This helps keep the tension throughout the entire body and not just in the legs and feet.

(8)

As you develop your routine, use enough variety in step patterns and gesturing (arms, head, shoulders, hips, etc.) patterns to keep the dance interesting as well as challenging.

(9)

To determine if your dance is challenging enough (high-intensity level, fast tempo, and sufficient duration), check your pulse after doing the dance and see if you have reached your training zone and are at your steady state.

(10)

If a particular step pattern or gesture is difficult to learn or remember, change it. You can always modify or change any part of your own dance or anyone else's to fit your own needs and abilities.

(11)

You have a repertoire of gestures and step patterns as explained in Chapter 5. Use these for starters if you like, and then add your own. There are so many different combinations.

(12)

As the tempo of your music increases your dance steps to a faster tempo, you need to take smaller steps and use less space. This enables you to stay with the beat of the music. For example, you do a slide and you cover three feet of space with each slide. As you put the slide to fast music, you only have time enough to cover one foot of space. Your slide will need to be smaller to fit the music and to allow you to keep on the beat.

(13)

Be sure that you determine the underlying or steady beat of the music. (This can be accomplished by clapping or writing down each beat as explained later in this chapter.) This will determine how easy you will be able to choreograph and perform to it. Count the underlying beats in sets of four or eight if possible. (Most music that you'll choose will be in $\frac{4}{4}$ time to make this counting possible.)

(14)

If you have difficulty with tempo or phrasing or in finding the underlying beat, it would be best to find another song or version of the same song.

(15)

Choreograph to the sets of four or eight beats rather than to the melody. The only time that the melody or overlying beat is important to choreographing is when it repeats itself and you wish to do the same step sequence each time. For example, you can dance the same step pattern each time the chorus is repeated in the song.

(16)

After you have determined your step patterns, decide how many times you will repeat the step pattern. The routines in the book repeat the same step patterns two, four, eight, or sixteen times. You want to repeat just enough to make the dance easier to remember. If you have too many repetitions it will become boring to dance.

⑰

Start each new step sequence with the right foot to make the transition smoother. Very seldom do you need to start with the left foot. You want the transitions smooth and continuous so that your pulse rate stays at your steady state.

⑱

After writing the step sequences down on paper, mentally go through the dance as you listen to the music.

⑲

Once you have the step patterns sequenced and are able to coordinate them with the music, then coordinate the arms or other gestures with your steps. (Gestures are defined as the movement of any non-weight-bearing body part.)

⑳

Remember — you are choreographing an aerobic dance, not a dance to be performed for an audience. Make sure that you execute the steps and gestures with lots of tension (firmness). A relaxed, easy style may be fine for an audience to enjoy, but it won't work the heart enough to give you the proper training effect.

SUGGESTIONS FOR MOVEMENT PATTERNS

Suggestions for movement patterns that will help you choreograph routines are as follows:

LOCOMOTOR ACTIVITIES

Movement that carries the body from one place to another through space.

- Walking
- Jogging
- Running
- Sliding
- Galloping
- Rocking
- Marching
- Prancing
- Leaping
- Jumping — there are five basic jumps. They are:

  Take-off   Landing
  One foot to the same foot (also called a hop)
  One foot to the other foot (called a leap)
  One foot to two feet (called a stride)
  Two feet to two feet
  Two feet to one foot

NON-LOCOMOTOR ACTIVITIES

Movement performed over a stationary base.

- Bending
- Stretching
- Curling
- Twisting
- Gesturing
- Turning
- Pushing
- Pulling
- Opening
- Closing
- Swinging (arms, legs, torso)
- Swaying
- Kicking (from the ankle, knee, hip)

BODY SHAPES
- Straight or angular
- Widespread
- Round
- Twisted
- Symmetrical
- Asymmetrical

FORCE
- Heavy
- Light
- Gradually
- Suddenly

DIRECTIONALITY
- Up
- Down
- Right side
- Left side
- Forward
- Back

PATHWAYS
- Curved (i.e., circle, figure 8)
- Straight
- Combinations of straight and curved
- Diagonal (i.e., zig zags)

LEVELS
(of the body as well as different body parts)
- Low
- Medium
- High

SPEED

- Fast
- Slow
- Gradually
- Suddenly

EXTENSIONS OF DIFFERENT BODY PARTS

- Arms
- Hands
- Legs
- Upper torso

DANCE STEPS

- Polka
- Charleston
- Cha-cha
- Grapevine
- Schottische
- Two-step
- Jitterbug
- Disco step
- Foxtrot
- Hustle

DANCES

- Mexican hat dance
- Bunny hop (an American line dance)
- Hora (Israeli folk dance)
- Square dancing

COMBINING STEPS AND BEATS

As you begin choreographing your aerobic dances, keep the steps simple. First, try four steps and keep repeating them. For example:

- **Jog,** 16 times — 16 counts
- **Hop kick,** 4 times — 8 counts
- **Rock,** 16 times — 16 counts
- **Jump,** 8 times — 8 counts

} 48 counts

You have a forty-eight count sequence that you can keep repeating throughout the song you have chosen.

Put these steps with your **underlying beats.**

/ / / / / / / / = 8 beats
Jog each beat = 8 times

/ / / / / / / / = 8 beats
Jog each beat = 8 times

/ / / / / / / / = 8 beats
Hop kick (takes 2 beats at a time) = 4 times

/ / / / / / / / = 8 beats
Rock each beat = 8 times

/ / / / / / / / = 8 beats
Rock each beat = 8 times

/ / / / / / / / = 8 beats
Jump each beat = 8 times

Now it wouldn't be very interesting or enjoyable to keep repeating this forty-eight count sequence standing in one place, so look at the different aspects of movement and decide ways in which you can make the forty-eight count sequence more fun and challenging to learn and perform.

For example:

- Jog, 8 times, forward; jog, 8 times, backward.
- Hop and kick diagonally alternating feet, 4 times (ie., hop right, kick left leg to diagonal right; hop left, kick right leg to diagonal left).
- Rock forward and backward, 4 times; rock right side to left side, 4 times.
- Jump, 4 times, turning right, completing a circle; jump, 4 times, turning left, completing a circle.

Now add gestures to your sequence:

- Jog with arms at side (above the waist) using jogger's arms (Chapter 5).
- Hop kick with arms shoulder height, straight, straight to the side.
- Rock with arms in same position as in the hop kick.
- Jump with arms raised straight above your shoulders.

Pull all this together with your music and enjoy!

As you begin to feel comfortable with your choreographing, add more steps to your sequence to increase the challenge. The next progression would be to plan two different sequences for a more interesting dance. With your favorite music and your enjoyable, vigorous routines, you're on your way to developing your own aerobic dance program.

9
UNDERSTANDING BODY COMPOSITION AND WEIGHT CONTROL

"As a man advances in life
he gets what is better than
admiration — judgment
to estimate things at their own value."

Samuel Johnson

For all those persons who are interested in making change or an improvement — especially in their "outer" appearance — this chapter should be thought-provoking.

We all will admit to the fact that we'd like to remain healthy forever! If we take care of the body we have, it should, in return, provide us with a comfortable life. We acknowledge the fact that we want our heart, lungs, and blood vessels to function well to provide for this comfortable life. But, unfortunately, we can't **see** our heart, lungs, and blood vessels. It thus becomes a rather abstract lifelong aerobic goal of enjoying relevant **secondary** benefits.

Many individuals will, therefore, initially focus on the **concrete** form of their understanding of "fitness" when it comes to improvement for themselves — something that we can **directly see.** Thus, since you can see when your body looks nice, lean, and toned — and likewise, when it looks "out of shape", flabby, and full of fat deposits — you tend to want to change those aspects that involve **immediate** feedback — the outward physical appearance. As previously mentioned, this outer appearance is not the major importance of true fitness, for we can live without well-toned muscles or a trim figure (but we can't live long without a good strong heart and lungs). Nevertheless, accompanying facets to your fitness program are feeling and looking nice, being strong, and staying well. Since we can directly and concretely **see** these qualities, let's size up what each of us have to "work with" and set some attainable goals for ourselves.

REALISTIC SELF-APPRAISAL

In order to understand what **our** best outer physical appearance can be, we must first recognize and **accept** our very makeup. At

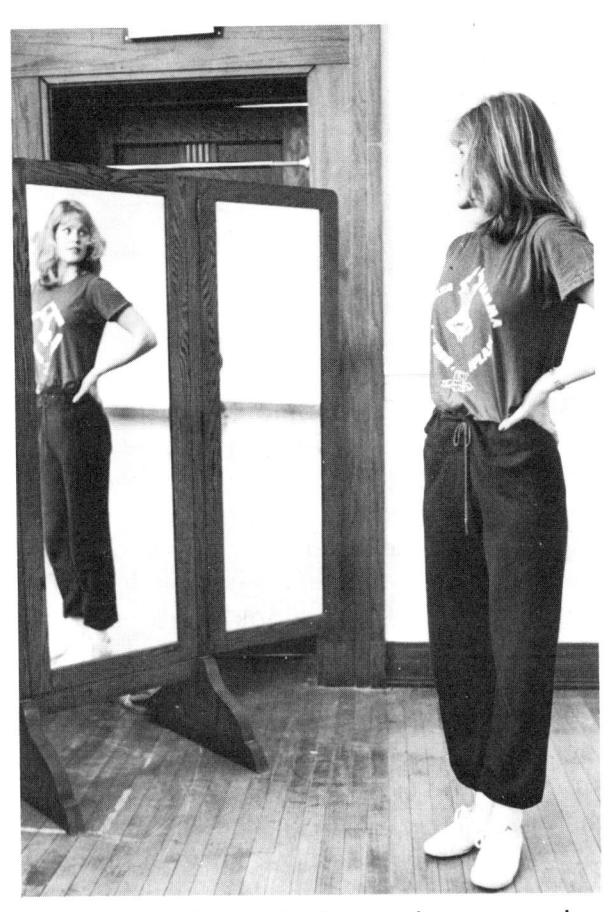

In order to understand what our best outer physical appearance can be, we must first recognize and accept our very makeup.

conception we were all blessed with a specific genetic makeup for which we can thank our parents! We each possess a specific body type (physical classification of the human body), and we can never be the size and shape of someone whom we idolize — be that person smaller or bigger than we are! If we start out with a similar body type, we may be able to come close, but there is no use wishing that we were 6 feet, 2 inches tall when we are 4 feet, 11 inches, for we basically cannot change our inherent structure. Likewise, to desire to look like a twig when we're built like a tree trunk is not being realistic.

Sheldon[1] differentiates between body types and accompanying characteristics (extremes) as follows. Which do you seem to be most like?

①

Endomorphy — roundness and softness of the body. Features of this type:

- Short neck
- High square shoulders
- Large abdomen over thorax
- Breasts developed
- Round full buttocks
- Skin is soft and smooth

②

Mesomorphy — square body with hard, rugged, and prominent muscles. Features:

- Large bones covered with thick muscle
- Forearm thickness, heavy wrist, hands, and fingers
- Slender waist
- Broad shoulders
- Trunk upright

③

Ectomorphy — linearity, fragility and delicacy of body. Features:

- Small bones
- Thin muscles
- Shoulders droop; not much muscularity
- Long limbs and short trunk (not necessarily a tall person, though)
- No bulging muscles anywhere
- Shoulder blades tend to wing out in back

Once we begin to realize that we are each a specific body type, we can then begin to understand a second component of our self-appraisal. This is understanding what then makes up our body mass, or "body composition."

UNDERSTANDING BODY COMPOSITION

Your body is composed of two weights: **lean weight** and **fat weight.** Lean weight is composed of your bones, muscles, and internal organs. Fat weight is just that. It is that **stored energy** that you are wearing for future use. The amount of each that you carry is important to know to understand what is best for your **heart's** best health.

Your lean weight declines (weighs less) after maturity (when you stop growing) at a certain steady pace every year. This is one of the beautiful aging processes. To slow down the aging processes and maintain your strength, you need to incorporate muscular strength and endurance as part of your total fitness program. Basically, the only portion of your **lean** weight that you can greatly change (for the better) is your **muscle** weight. It's rather difficult to attempt to increase lean weight by making your bones heavier or by increasing the size of your liver! (Remember — lean weight equals bones, muscles, and internal organs.) You can, however, increase your lean weight through a muscle-thickening program called strength training or weight training. Since thicker (denser) muscle fiber weighs more, your lean weight will increase.

For each individual's amount of lean, then, a certain percentage of fat can be "worn" to maintain ideal cardiorespiratory efficiency. Body fat has several necessary functions:

①

To provide storage for the fat-soluble vitamins A, D, K, and E. (The other vitamins are water soluble, and if they are not used daily as taken in, they are excreted through the urine, etc.)

②

To insulate the body from the weather.

③

To protect the internal organs from shocks and blows delivered to the body, i.e., falls, physical contact, etc.

④

To provide the storage of future energy (go-power).

Beyond supplying these needs, we just **don't need** the extra weight and stress that fat places on the heart.

An appropriate percentage of fat to be worn with the lean is approximately 20 to 22 percent body fat for women and 10 to 12½ percent body fat for men. Women carry a higher percentage of fat because an extra layer of fat is present below the skin, and because breast tissue is primarily fat. But if we wear more fat tissue than the suggested amounts above, it simply adds additional risk factors associated with heart disease. If we wear **less** than the above ideal percentage it **doesn't matter, UNLESS:**

- We are malnourishing ourselves
- We cosmetically wish to look heavier

For instance, endurance athletes, like marathon runners or Olympic gymnasts, do not carry the suggested ideal percentage. They carry much less. They simply burn it off and don't carry the excess. They (usually) eat right to provide the necessary nutrients and energy and thus display a firm, trim, toned look. The wobbly-fat, "gelatin" look is absent from these extremely physical people, and yet they stay well.

In contrast are the anorexic individuals (persons who exhibit the starvation disease, anorexia nervosa). They also may carry **less** than the suggested ideal percentage of body fat and accomplish this feat through a process of **also eliminating their lean weight.** They desire a trim look but go about it in a way that is against all physiological principles of proper weight loss. To them, weight loss means purely dropping pounds to be slim at all costs, no matter what kind of weight it is, fat **or** lean. This is an **extremely detrimental** way to lose weight!

To enable individuals to understand **healthy** slimness and **unhealthy** slimness, an in-depth look at weight control follows later in this chapter.

DETERMINING YOUR BODY COMPOSITION

There is no way in which to determine the amount of body fat and body lean that a person has merely by looking at the person. An assessment of body composition involves determining as precisely as possible, an individual's body fat and lean body weight. Such an assessment allows an **accurate estimate** to be made of what an individual's **ideal weight should be.** This is important, since the traditional approach of using standardized weight

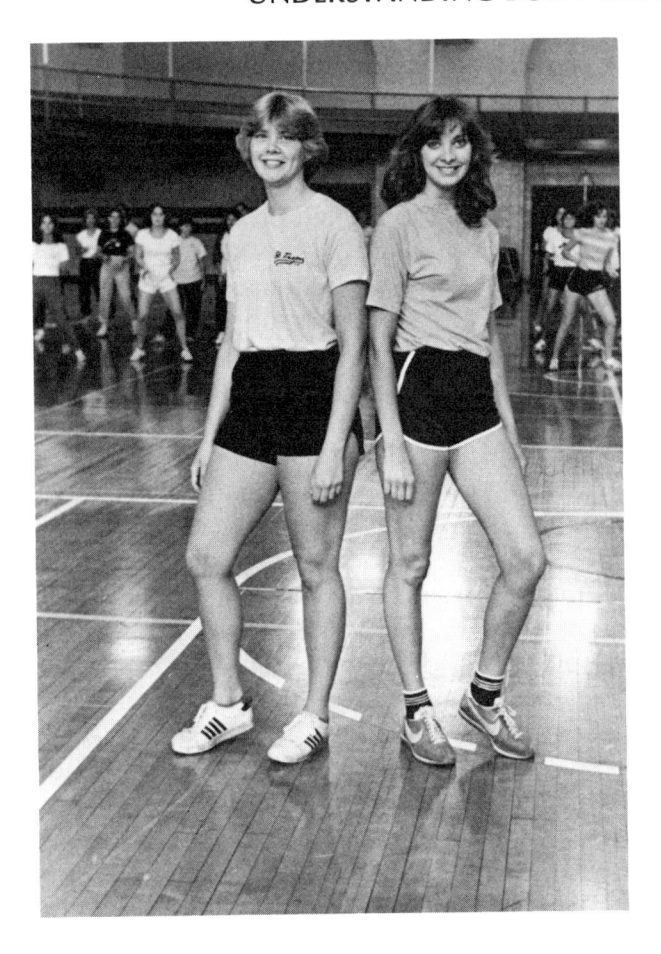

It is impossible to determine "ideal weight" just by looking at someone. The amount of lean weight that you have determines what *fat* weight you should wear with that lean, and only then can *your* individual "ideal weight" be determined. Both of these college women are approximately 5'10" tall and are carrying the same percentage of body fat (28%) on their individual leans. At left, Paula's ideal weight is 145. On the right, Jill's ideal weight is 114. Ideal weight is calculated with the use of a scale and a skinfold caliper or an underwater weighing tank.

tables adjusted for sex, height, and frame size has been shown to be grossly inaccurate for a rather large percentage of the population. The ideal weight within any one category of these tables can vary up to twenty-two pounds. It is not unusual for an individual to fall within the normal range for his or her category but to actually have ten to thirty pounds of excess body fat![2]

Consequently, measurement techniques have been sought which will more accurately determine whether an individual is overweight (overfat) or obese and then quantify exactly by how much. Several excellent techniques are available:

- Measuring skinfold thickness
- Underwater weighing (specific gravity)
- Using both skinfold thickness and anthropometric measures of bone thickness and/or girth measurements

Because of ease of use in an aerobic dance setting and availability of equipment, only the first technique will be described in detail here, although underwater weighing will be covered briefly.

MEASURING SKINFOLD THICKNESS

There are a number of skinfold measurement formulas that use various sites on the body for calculations. A formula that we prefer to use for aerobic dance class purposes was developed by Dr. Jack H. Wilmore, then of the University of California at Davis. According to Wilmore[3], lean body weight, relative percent fat, and relative weights for an individual can be accurately measured by the following formula, which has a coefficient of correlation of .90 — .93 r. In mathematical terminology, this means that it is a quite accurate measurement tool for persons aged eighteen through thirty-five who are not extremely obese. The three steps to this procedure are:

UNDERSTANDING BODY COMPOSITION AND WEIGHT CONTROL

①

Step 1 determines how much lean weight (bones, muscles, and organs) you have, **in pounds.**

②

Step 2 determines the **percentage** of fat that you are carrying along with your lean weight. You can thus place yourself in a category of relative percent fat (the ratio of fat to fat-free weight). The four categories described here are "obesity," "overweight," "ideal weight," and "underfat weight."

③

Step 3, then, determines **relative weights for you** by giving you your pound weights (when you step on a scale) for the four categories described. You are then able to realize how much fat weight, in pounds, you need to lose, gain, or maintain to be at the ideal percentage of fat to lean, and therefore at your **ideal weight.** It thus gives you concrete numbers with which to set goals. Rather than the abstract thought, "I think I need to lose twenty-five pounds," you can say with assurance to yourself "I need to lose eighteen to twenty-one pounds of body fat at my present lean weight."

ONGOING, LIFETIME ASSESSMENT

To initiate this procedure today, or at any future date, an individual needs only to have access to two accurate measurement tools:
- A "doctor's" scale to determine the present accurate nude weight, in pounds
- A calibrated, precision instrument called a "skinfold caliper," which will determine the present skinfold thickness, in millimeters. (Incidentally, the inexpensive plastic-type devices available are about as accurate as using your index finger, thumb, and a ruler, and pinching an inch!) You are interested in **accuracy,** so use a precision instrument made by a reputable company.

UNDERWATER WEIGHING TECHNIQUE

After middle age, body density changes, and the aforementioned procedure becomes a less accurate tool, especially for **inactive** people. A more accurate body composition assessment for older persons (or for persons of any age for that matter), then, is the underwater weighing technique. Underwater weighing requires a special facility with a water tank and a submersible scale that the individual sits upon. Specific gravity is determined (ratio of the density of the person to the density of the water). Since an object immersed in a fluid loses an amount of weight equivalent to the weight of the fluid that is displaced[4], and since the density of the object is two and one-half times greater than the density of water[5], an individual's specific gravity can be determined. A figure can then be calculated to represent the percentage of fat that the subject currently has. All of the above configurations tell an individual the correct amount of lean weight, the percentage of fat currently present, and the ideal weight toward which the individual should work (if not presently there).

WHAT DO THE CATEGORIES MEAN?

Visually, in terms of a traffic light, "obesity" is the red light — **STOP NOW** and think what all this extra fat is doing to your cardiorespiratory

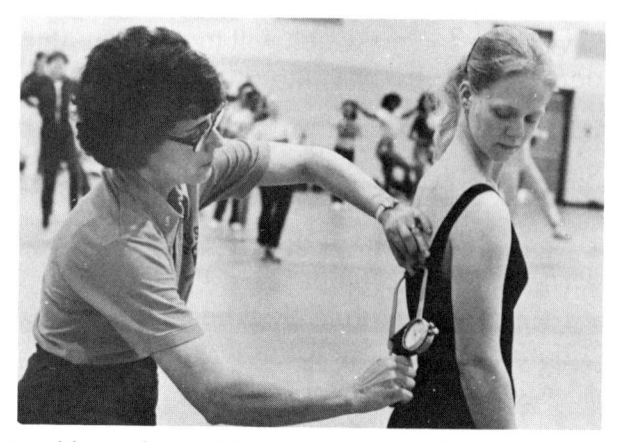

A calibrated, precision instrument called a skinfold caliper determines the present skinfold thickness, in millimeters.

health. "Obesity" describes when a woman is 30 percent (or more) body fat and a man is 20 percent (or more) body fat to the amount of lean that they are carrying. If lean weight increases (due to a weight training program, etc.), the percentage of fat worn with that lean will go up, i.e., your ideal weight would go up. But, since your lean weight **declines** as you age, the ideal weight declines because you want to wear still 20 to 22 percent fat (women) or 10 to 12½ percent fat (men) on that declining lean. Therefore, your ideal weight usually decreases with age. If you remain the same weight as when you were first married, thirty years ago, you have usually gained extra **fat** weight. Because your activity level and metabolism both slow down with age, increasing your exercise and decreasing your food intake will assist you with your ongoing lifetime assessment process.

"Overweight" is the yellow light, "caution" category. Beware! You are in the category where many Americans are finding themselves today — creeping overfatness. Since you are "overfat," you need to be aware of your intake and output of energy (eating and exercising). For women, it's 25 to 29 percent body fat, and for men it's 15 to 19 percent body fat.

"Ideal weight" is the "go" for it three-pound range of your current lean weight wearing a specific proper percentage of fat. For women it is 20 to 22 percent fat and for men it's 10 to 12½ percent fat. Your ideal weight changes in proportion to your lean weight change(s).

"Underfat" depicts the individual who is carrying less than the suggested ideal percentage of body fat to the amount of lean that he/she has. Again, it doesn't matter how underfat you are, as long as you eat right and don't malnourish your body.

Thus, with the aforementioned formula (and there are other excellent ones to use), you can, on a continual, lifetime basis, assess the ideal weight for your **heart's** best health.

"If we were all nudists we'd stay in better shape."[7]

John Derek

WEIGHT CONTROL

Weight control = controlling the amount of body fat that you carry. Nine out of ten women and men who are currently students of aerobic dance at the university and community in which we teach desire to lose weight.[8] And, following skinfold testing of this group, it was found that 91 percent **need** to lose weight in the form of body fat!

The average percentage of body fat exhibited by women entering an aerobic dance course has been 27 percent.[9] No significant data have been collected on men due to the relatively small number enrolled thus far. Of those who have, however, the average percentage of body fat exhibited has been 16 percent. (Each quarter/semester, the number of men enrolling in the course doubles or triples. We predict in two years the ratio of men to women will be 50/50!)

The principles of weight control include **weight maintenance** (staying the same composition of fat to the amount of lean you're carrying), **weight gain** (almost always in terms of lean weight gain, not fat weight gain), and **weight loss** (always in terms of loss of body fat).

WEIGHT MAINTENANCE

This refers to the fact that

- Your current composition of fat to lean is ideal for your cardiovascular best health
- You are pleased with how you look (cosmetically)
- You have enough strength to function well in your daily life of work and recreation, to whatever extreme that may encompass. In order to remain at this constant weight, your **energy** must be in balance, i.e.:

"calories in" = "calories out"
(eating)   = (expenditure; exercise)

Since a decline in "calories out" occurs with aging (your metabolism slows down and you are less active), a decline in "calories in" (eat less) must accompany the aging processes.

WEIGHT GAIN

This almost always refers to the gaining of lean tissue, or the thickening of muscle fiber. When you want to cosmetically look better, or to have an increased amount of strength for a sport or for daily needs, weight training is the type of activity in which to engage. Since you would be using more energy in a day than you did prior to the weight training program, you would need to "calories in" (eat) the **same** amount as you are newly expending (in the form of "calories out") with weight training, for maintenance. However, to **gain lean** and **lose extra body fat** simultaneously requires you to **eat less** while providing the **increased exercise** of weight training. Only if you are at ideal weight or underfat weight should you accompany this weight-gain program with an increase in caloric intake.[10]

Weight gain would then directly mean an increase in muscle mass, or thickening those "rubber bands" that you have as muscles! Thicker rubber bands (i.e., muscles) are more dense and weigh more than thin rubber bands. You primarily do not gain more muscle cells — you thicken what you presently have.

WEIGHT LOSS

This always refers to the **purposeful** losing of **fat weight** — never lean weight. Weight loss, of course, can occur to both your lean and your fat according to how you go about losing the weight. The director of the local Better Business Bureau has stated that one of the top two frauds with which he comes in contact is weight loss products and information. "People will do *anything* to lose weight. You would be amazed at the amount of fraud that is being perpetrated on the American public. If it's easy, people will try it! If you want to get rich quick, go into the weight loss business."[11] This last statement was, of course, spoken in jest but is, sadly, very true. Before you spend your money on **any** claim, product, device, or book, call your local Better Business Bureau. However, if you understand the principles of weight loss, you will always be able to determine a product's (program's, etc.) worth before you spend money, time, and energy on it.

A CASE STUDY ON WEIGHT-LOSS PRODUCT USE

A student who had been skinfold tested at the onset of a ten-week aerobic dance course requested our input on a weight-loss product that she (the student) was planning to use. The label stated that the product is to be consumed three times a day for one month. No other food is taken in. (The product is a powder in a can and is to be mixed with liquid.) It provides all the nutrients needed daily. It is recommended that exercise not accompany the use of the product. At the end of one month, when you have lost a substantial amount of weight, you eat regular meals again. Five pages of accompanying research (that comes with the product) state that the product will cause you to lose only fat weight and not lean, and quotes by various physicians worldwide claim the product's authenticity.

After much discussion with both a resident physiologist and a nutrition specialist who attempted to encourage the student against the product's use, the student still took the powder. Approximately three weeks later, the student said that she had lost twelve pounds and requested a second skinfold test. Of the twelve pounds of weight loss, **eight pounds were lean** and four were fat! She was totally crushed that this new "miracle" product was assisting her in losing primarily her lean weight — rapidly.

A key lesson was learned early in life for this nineteen-year-old woman. Not only did she lose a substantial amount of lean weight, but when she begins to eat normally again, she will more than likely gain weight, **all of which will be fat** (if no strength training is incorporated).

PRINCIPLES OF WEIGHT LOSS (i.e., FAT LOSS)

①

Fat weight is the only kind of weight to lose. When a product claims to "get rid of excess body fluids," it's a joke! Body fluids are **not fat!** (Incidently, unnatural water retention, or "edema," is a condition to be monitored and treated by a doctor, not by your self-prescribed procedures or products.)

②

If you lose water weight (fluids) by sweating during exercise, you will, and should, gain it back in twenty-four hours to maintain your body's beautifully synchronized chemical balance. The energy-producing (metabolic) processes perform best when all of the necessary components are present. So don't be misled into believing that dropping your **water** weight is effective weight loss. It is part of your fat-free weight and is a vital part of your continuous well-being. You can understand, then, why weighing yourself **after** a strenuous exercise session is an inaccurate time to weigh.

③

Fat is metabolized more readily and efficiently by performing high- (or low-) intensity exercise for a **long duration of time.** If you are fit to work at the upper end of your training zone (i.e., high intensity) for thirty to forty-five minutes, you will have provided yourself with the most physiologically sound way to metabolize (burn off) that unwanted body fat.

> Endurance exercise depends on fuel being furnished to the muscles and liquid fat — cholesterol and triglycerides — is a far more important fuel than carbohydrates. Any exercise that lasts longer than 30 minutes has got to be nourished by liquid fat . . . Muscles burn fat directly — scientists thought that carbohydrates were the main fuel. That's only partially true. Carbohydrates are quickly exhausted. After 15 minutes of exercise, fat is burning and after 30 minutes the nutrition is almost wholly fat — the same fat that has been clogging the arteries of the cardiovascular system.[12]

The conclusion to one research study at the University of Illinois is that **you need to exercise for more than thirty minutes at a time to make significant changes in the fat content of the body.**

Wearing rubber suits, see-through plastic wrap around body parts, and on hot days heavy, long-sleeved "sweats," nylons, or tights, will tend to inhibit the free flow of sweat and will disallow it to perform its function of **cooling you.** When it is hot and humid, wear as little as possible when performing aerobics. You cannot metabolize (burn up) fat faster by increasing your body temperature through the wearing of more clothes!

④

Fat will metabolize off your body in a **general** way. You can't "spot reduce"! Spot reducing is perhaps the most prevalent misconception concerning fat weight loss and the one by which many unscrupulous people are defrauding unsuspecting overfat Americans out of millions of dollars every year.

By your genetic constitution, your body will use up its stored energy (fat) any way in which it is programmed to do so. You cannot do fifty leg lifts a day and hope to reduce the fat deposits in that area. You will shape up (thicken) the muscle fiber in the area — and toned muscles contain more of the enzymes involved in breaking down fat — but you do not burn off the fat there, or at any one particular location, necessarily. As energy is needed, it is withdrawn — first from the immediate sources — and when this is used up, it is withdrawn randomly from more permanent storage. It is then converted to an immediate usable form. Thus, you may lose weight in places you don't necessarily wish to at first, like your face, breast area, etc. But with a little perseverance, you'll metabolize off the fat in those "problem" areas, too.

⑤

Fat weight loss is most readily accomplished through a **combined** program **of diet and exercise.** It is very difficult to lose fat weight by only exercising more, and **not** changing your eating habits (less "calories in"). And, when you **only diet** (eat less food) and step on a scale, the weight loss **is not all fat.** According to the way in which you have dieted, your weight loss is approximately one-half to two-thirds (50 to 68 percent) fat loss and one-third to one-half (33 to 50 percent) lean weight loss.

And if your life-style and habits (of eating and exercising) don't change, after you stop "dieting" and you gain back your lost weight, **what you gain back is all fat.** You are therefore worse off! You lose both fat and lean and regain back only fat. Over a lifetime of this "yo-yo" crash dieting, you can see how you are detrimentally changing your entire body composition.

When you diet (eat less) and exercise (expend more calories or energy), you tend to lose approximately 100 percent fat. This is the only kind of weight that you want to lose. And exercise speeds weight loss, not only by burning calories while you're working out, but also by revitalizing your metabolism so that you **continue** to burn calories more readily for the next few hours.

⑥

You can both gain weight and lose weight with an endurance exercise program. You will be metabolizing off fat for energy (loss) and building up muscle (gain) simultaneously. So if you do not realize a change on the scale immediately, don't be disappointed!

⑦

A **light** exercise program will **increase** your appetite, and a **strenuous** exercise program will **decrease** your appetite. You will find that after an endurance aerobic hour, your desire for food greatly diminishes. You will have time to carefully select, or prepare, what you know is good for you, rather than ravenously grab that easy, high-calorie junk food just sitting around.

⑧

It is easier to eat less food than it is to exercise it off. Consider the following for a 120-to 130-pound person:

- It takes approximately two minutes to walk off (two steps per second) one potato chip (ten calories).
- It takes five minutes of high-intensity aerobic dancing (eight calories per minute times five minutes = forty calories) to a fast-tempoed song to dance off (a bite) one-sixth of a candy bar that contains 240 calories.
- In most aerobic dance sessions you will only burn about 300 calories. So think twice about rewarding yourself with high-calorie treats afterward if you are seriously interested in losing your fat weight. Instead, replenish your water loss with no-calorie, yet quite filling, ice water.

⑨

Since there is no such thing as a constipated endurance aerobic dancer, you will, with regularity, eliminate your solid wastes. Regular, rhythmic stimulation of the entire digestion and elimination processes will be one of the side benefits that you'll not necessarily talk about but for which you will certainly be glad!

⑩

And, the basic bottom-line principle for fat weight loss is: the body's energy balance determines whether or not a person gains or loses body fat. Two words — how very simple it all is. And yet look at all of the products, devices, and books that people buy to find the magic easy way. There simply is no magic — just **self-discipline** to understand that energy is the basis for change and will result in a proper weight loss if less caloric energy is intaken and more caloric energy is expended.

CALORIC INTAKE AND USE

Everything that you eat or drink becomes "you" for either a short or lengthy duration of time. Thus, you are what you eat! This means that the food nutrients you eat are used to maintain basic body functions such as breathing, blood circulation, normal body temperature, and growth and repair of all tissue, and are related to fixed factors such as age, body size, and physiological state. Any kind of caloric intake that your body doesn't use or doesn't eliminate through solid or liquid waste is kept and "worn" as body fat for future energy needs. Thus, if you don't **use** it, or **eliminate** it, you **wear** it!

UNDERSTANDING BODY COMPOSITION AND WEIGHT CONTROL

CALORIC EXPENDITURE

Every moment of every day, no matter what activity you are engaged in — from sleeping to aerobic dancing — you are using up calories. Caloric energy expenditure is most influenced by your life-style — how physically active you are all day. The body's basic needs are more or less fixed, but the amount of physical exertion in which an individual engages is a personal decision. How physically active a person's life is depends on choice of profession (an aerobic dance instructor usually has more opportunities for vigorous physical exercise than a school bus driver or a college dean) and choice of recreational activities (playing cards requires fewer calories than leisurely walking).

It all depends upon a multitude of day-to-day choices: whether to walk to the local store or drive the car; use the stairs or elevator; rake the leaves or hire it done; go out for a bicycle ride after supper or watch a TV show. **How physically active a person's life is depends as much on attitude as it does on opportunity.**[13]

MAINTAINING YOUR WEIGHT

If you can picture this "energy in" and "energy out" in balance, you can then understand maintenance, or staying the same weight. For in order to remain at the same weight, you must intake (eat) the amount of calories you expend (burn up) every day.

How much energy do you eat and expend every day to stay at your current weight? (This needs to be established first.) To answer this, you need to determine two criteria:

- How much do you currently weigh? (a number in pounds)
- How active are you? Dr. Kenneth Cooper, in his book *The Aerobics Way*,[14] states that this number is determined by your life-style:

12 = sedentary: desk job, or constant studying, reading only leisure, park close to where you're going, take the elevators instead of stairs, TV watch instead of any physical type exertion in evenings, etc.

15 = active: walk to classes, ride bikes for recreation and errands, involved in an activity class or two every week, work out on your own, park far away and walk to your office, take the stairs, etc., enjoy "programming" exercise into your schedule as much as possible.

18 = pregnant and lactating women.

20 = manual labor job, varsity endurance twelve-month athlete who performs regular high-intensity work; the extremely physical life-style.

Directions:
Multiply your present weight times your life-style of activity (number is at the left margin of each description). The number you arrive at is the approximate number of calories you eat daily to maintain your current weight.

| PRESENT WEIGHT × TYPE OF LIFE-STYLE | =

| THE NUMBER OF CALORIES PER DAY YOU EAT TO STAY AT YOUR WEIGHT. |

Figure your numbers here:

_____ × _____ = _____

If you wish to **gain** weight, you must then **eat more** calories than this number.

If you wish to **lose** weight, you must then **eat less** calories than this number.

CALORIC INTAKE NEEDED TO GAIN LEAN WEIGHT

The caloric requirement to add one pound of body muscle is 2,500 calories. Thus, the

78 UNDERSTANDING BODY COMPOSITION AND WEIGHT CONTROL

daily caloric excess, over your maintenance number just figured, is 360 calories.[15]

1 pound of muscle gain	=	2,500 calories equivalent of 1 pound of muscle	÷	7 days in a week	=	360 daily excess calories to eat, over maintenance intake number

You must first, however, be at or below your ideal weight to go on an excess calorie eating program to gain muscle. You want to use your excess body fat, first, for your energy requirements.

Note: Intaking calories greater than 1,000 per day *over* the number needed to maintain weight is, however, likely to result in weight gain as body fat, even if you are exercising strenuously on a regular basis.[16]

CALORIC INTAKE NEEDED TO LOSE BODY FAT

It is physiologically impossible to lose more than two to three pounds of body fat per week.[17] A weight loss greater than this will represent water and lean body tissue. (You'll look lousy, feel weak, be hard to live with, will inherit every germ floating by you, etc., when you drop your **lean** weight.)

To systematically drop that unwanted extra body fat, you need to **drop 3,500 calories** a week (or 500 per day) **to lose one pound of body fat** and **7,000 calories** a week (or 1,000 per day) **to lose two pounds** of body fat per week.

To lose:

1 pound fat	=	3,500 calories	÷	7 days per week	=	500 calories a day less than your maintenance number

To lose:

2 pounds fat	=	3,500 × 2 = 7,000 calories	÷	7 days per week	=	1,000 calories a day less than your maintenance number

Note: However, if you desire to drop two pounds a week, but the total calorie intake would be less than 1,200, you need to re-establish your goal and lose only one to one and a half pounds per week. **You never want to eat fewer than 1,200 calories per day.** A daily diet of less than 1,200 calories is likely to be deficient in needed nutrients for you to grow, repair, stay well, and have energy to perform daily tasks and leisure. (Sometimes on a one-to-one basis a doctor will prescribe a patient to eat fewer than 1,200 calories per day, but he or she will provide extensive guidelines and supplementation. This is **only** under strict supervision of a doctor's care.)

To lose one or two pounds of fat per week, the individual needs to then eliminate 500 or 1,000 calories every day. This reduction can be accomplished by either eating less or exercising more. But remember, for one hour of aerobic dance (including the warmup, aerobic dancing, cool down, and relaxation), you will only use up approximately 300 calories. Is it realistic to think that every day you will engage in two or three **more hours** of aerobics (than you now do)? It's highly unlikely for the average individual! Therefore, eliminating 500 or 1,000 calories should predominantly be **eating less food**. If you have yet to develop an aerobic fitness program, of course, your elimination of 500 or 1,000 calories per day would come from both the increased exercise (intensity and duration) **and** eating less food.

KNOW THYSELF

Taking time to educate yourself about your own body composition and about how to control your weight can be an interesting and rewarding experience. It will provide you

UNDERSTANDING BODY COMPOSITION AND WEIGHT CONTROL

with a basis of understanding how the human body physiologically works and how it **doesn't** work! You can then be alert to all of the false notions of weight loss that are rampant today, and you can develop a program that will work for **you**.

RECORDING WEIGHT MAINTENANCE, GAIN, AND LOSS

Chart VI has been provided to record your weight maintenance, loss, or gain for a ten-week period.

Directions:

①
Record your starting weight at zero area and where it states "starting weight," and "start of class weight."

②
Weigh once a week, first thing in the morning **after** arising, **after** elimination, and **before** you eat breakfast. This is the most accurate time of the day to weigh.

③
Record a maintenance weight in zero block line, initially. Maintenance — or staying the same — later on is recorded in the same block line as the previous week.

④
Record weight **gain** pounds as plus numbers of blocks **up** from the last recorded weight.

⑤
Record weight **loss** pounds **down** from the last recorded weight.

⑥
Record a final weight where it states "end of class weight."

⑦
Determine a final **total** maintenance gain or loss figure, where it states "+/- total: _____" weight for 10 week period.

Turn it in to the instructor the last week of class, if requested for a course.

10

PROPER DIET TO COMPLETE YOUR TOTAL FITNESS LOOK

*"Choose what is best;
habit will soon render it
agreeable and easy."*

Pythasoras

NUTRIENTS FOR "GOING" AND "GROWING"

Your body has two basic types of nutrient needs:

- Foods that keep you "going" — the energy needs
- Foods that keep you "growing" — the growth, repair, and regulation of body processes needs.

Nutrients are chemical substances that your body gets from food during the digestion process. About fifty nutrients are known to be needed by your body through your diet — "diet" here meaning **total intake of food and drink.** Essential nutrients are those that your body cannot make or is unable to make in adequate amounts. Therefore, they must be obtained from what you eat and drink. If they are not properly provided for in your diet, your body cannot perform well — mentally or physically.

IT IS YOUR CHOICE

Just as the opening quotation implies — **choose** what is best and **habit** will follow — **choice is a self-discipline that you must establish.** You might know what is "good-for-you" food and "junk" food, but if you don't then **eat** the best choice available, you really don't know good nutrition at all! Good health, optimum fitness, or good nutrition is not just knowing what is right, but **doing** it.

PROPER DIET TO COMPLETE YOUR TOTAL FITNESS LOOK

Good Choice

- A food or drink that provides the nutrients you need to go and grow.

"Junk" Food

- A food that is high in salt, fat, or sugar.

NUTRIENTS WORK TOGETHER IN TEAMS

The nutrients that your body needs can be grouped into the following six categories:

- Proteins
- Carbohydrates
- Fats
- Vitamins
- Minerals
- Water

When you provide all of these categories, each in the proper amounts (called "balancing your diet"), your body will perform like a finely tuned car or precision musical instrument. The movements and sounds could not be sweeter. However, when you decide to establish your own (usually misinformed) needs and priorities and overconsume some nutrients while underconsuming others, you are interfering with the body's balance.

If you know little about human physiology (how the body works), **don't** resort to just **any** source for what and how to eat well. There is an abundant quantity of excellent, easy-to-read, scientific literature that has been researched with controls and that will explain what balance of the above nutrients is needed. Read and follow information from established professionals rather than from movie stars or magazines on the supermarket racks. These people are interested in your money. Period.

SUPPLYING THE NEEDS

A well-balanced diet is one that contains the proper amounts of the six basic nutrients, established according to your age, sex, activity level, and state of wellness. Note the following:

- All persons need the same nutrients all their lives but in varying amounts.
- Larger amounts are needed for growth than for maintaining the body.
- Preadolescent children need smaller amounts of (food and) nutrients than adults, although they need the same ones.
- Boys and men need and use more nutrients and energy than girls and women.
- The only exception to the above is the need for iron. Women of childbearing age need more iron than other people.
- Active people require more nutrients that provide energy than inactive people.
- People recovering from illness need more nutrients than when in good health.[1]

These nutrients can be supplied by eating from the four food groups, as illustrated in the pamphlet "Guide to Good Eating, A Recommended Daily Pattern," published by the National Dairy Council.[2] It is not always possible to intake all essential nutrients every twenty-four hours. What **is** important is that over a span of several days and weeks there is a continual selection from the four groups to meet nutrient needs.

MILK GROUP

This is the only group that changes, according to servings you need, in reference to your age. Adults need two servings (except pregnant or lactating women, who need four servings); growing, preadolescent children need three servings; and teenagers need four servings. The nutrients involved are needed to build the basic structure and strength of bones and teeth, assist in the production of energy needs, and help in the growth and maintenance of every living cell.

One serving is equal to any of the following choices that you make:

1 cup milk (low fat milk has half the calories)
1 cup yogurt (yogurt is fermented milk)
1 cup pudding

82 PROPER DIET TO COMPLETE YOUR TOTAL FITNESS LOOK

milk Group

2 Servings/Adults
4 Servings/Teenagers
3 Servings/Children

Foods made from milk contribute part of the nutrients supplied by a serving of milk.

Calcium
Riboflavin (B$_2$)
Protein

Guide to Good Eating
A Recommended Daily Pattern

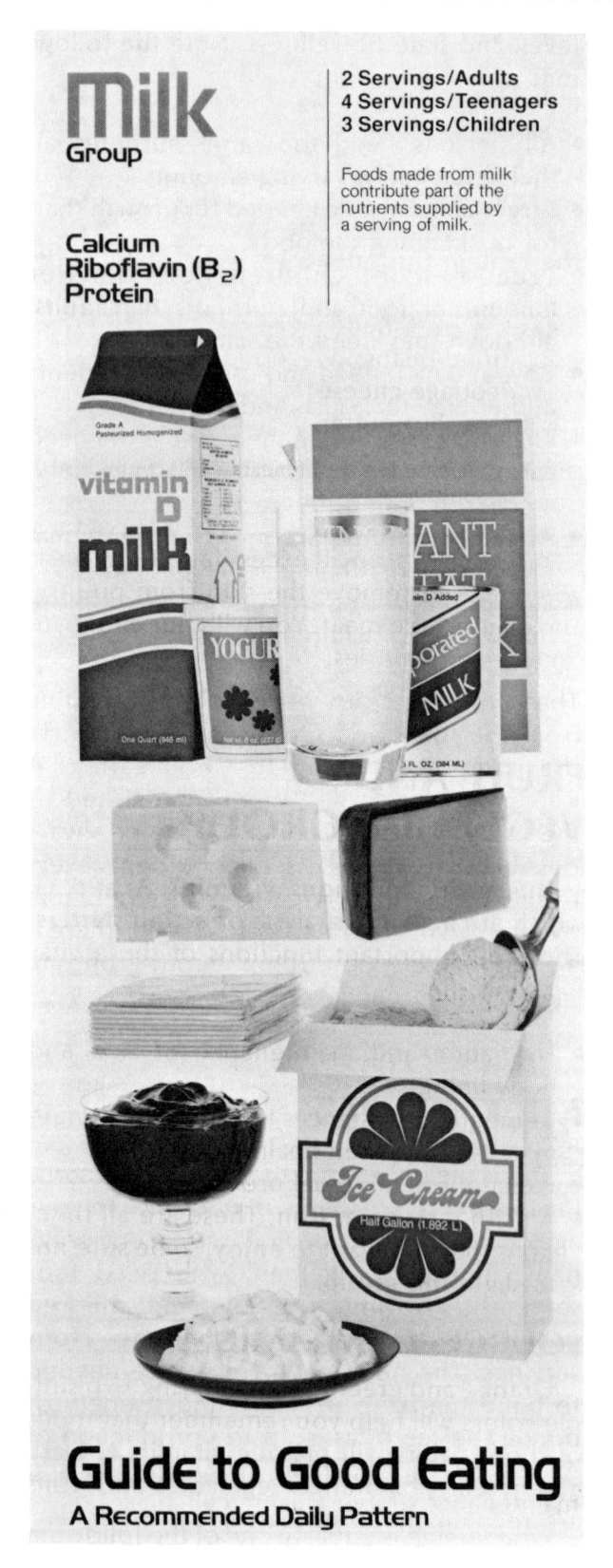

1½ slices (1½ oz.) cheddar cheese*
1¾ cup (2 big scoops) ice cream (It's **not** junk food!)
2 cups cottage cheese* (lowfat = fewer calories of energy intake).

*Count these cheeses as a serving of milk **or** meat group, but not both simultaneously.[3]

Remember — if you are not an avid "milk" fan, you can eat any of the food in the group and it will supply the calcium, riboflavin (B$_2$), and protein that you need.

MEAT GROUP

This group is called the "meat group," but there are also plant foods that, when eaten together, supply the needed protein, niacin, iron, and thiamin (B$_1$) and are then considered an alternative choice to eating meat.

Some of these plant foods that can be combined so that their proteins complement each other are: dried beans and whole wheat, dried beans and corn or rice, or peanuts and wheat.[4]

Make your own delicious mix of the following ingredients. It has a crunchy, slightly sweet, slightly salty taste. Purchase each item in one-pound lots (total cost is approximately twelve dollars), mix in a sixteen-quart container, and reseal the mixture in the airtight bags that each came in. Eating about one-half cup (snack) to one cup (a serving) a day provides an excellent tasting protein alternative that will last about six weeks. The cost immediately seems reasonable when you price even one steak! And, as a snack, it's much more nutritious and cheaper than the costly candy bars and fatty/salty snacks in bags.

Maz Mix

No salt or oil in process:
- Wheat nuts
- Sunflower seeds
- Almonds
- Pecans
- Walnuts (quartered)

PROPER DIET TO COMPLETE YOUR TOTAL FITNESS LOOK

Salted and oil in process:
- Dried soybeans
- Sesame sticks

Box each of:
- Chopped dates coated with oat flour
- Raisins

All persons need two servings per day of the Meat Group (except pregnant women, who need three servings per day).

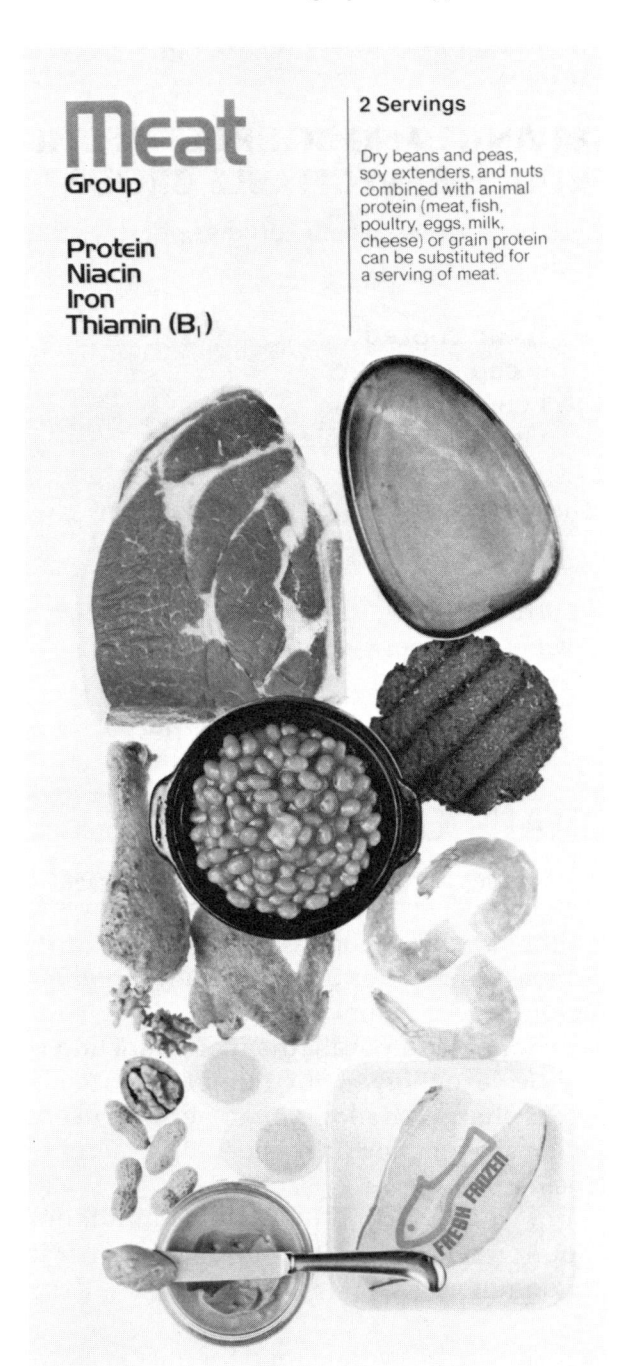

Meat Group

Protein
Niacin
Iron
Thiamin (B₁)

2 Servings

Dry beans and peas, soy extenders, and nuts combined with animal protein (meat, fish, poultry, eggs, milk, cheese) or grain protein can be substituted for a serving of meat.

One serving is equal to:

2 ounces cooked
 Lean meat
 Fish
 Poultry

OR

The Protein Equivalent:
2 eggs
2 slices (2 oz.) cheddar cheese*
1 cup dried beans; peas
½ cup cottage cheese*
4 Tbsp. peanut butter

*Count cheeses as serving of meat or milk, but not both simultaneously.[5]

Remember — strip all excess fat off any meat you eat. And remove the skin from poultry, and eat only the meat. You will thus eliminate unnecessary calories.

FRUIT AND VEGETABLE GROUP

This group provides vitamins A and C, which are actually catalysts or **action starters.** The most important functions of these vitamins include:

- Formation and maintenance of skin and body linings
- Cementing substances to promote strength in cells and hasten healing of injuries
- Functions in all visual processes
- Aids in the use of iron. These are all functions that you want to **enjoy,** so be sure not to slight this group.

SOURCES OF VITAMIN A

Orange and green. Remembering two simple colors will help you remember that foods of those colors will provide vitamin A. Dark green, leafy, or orange vegetables and fruits are recommended **at least** every other day. Because vitamin A is stored in the fat tissue of the body, an overdose intaken by supplementing this vitamin in pill form can be fatal. (The same is true for the other fat soluble vitamins: D, E, and K.)

Fruit-Vegetable Group

4 Servings

Vitamins A and C

Dark green, leafy, or orange vegetables and fruit are recommended 3 or 4 times weekly for vitamin A. Citrus fruit is recommended daily for vitamin C.

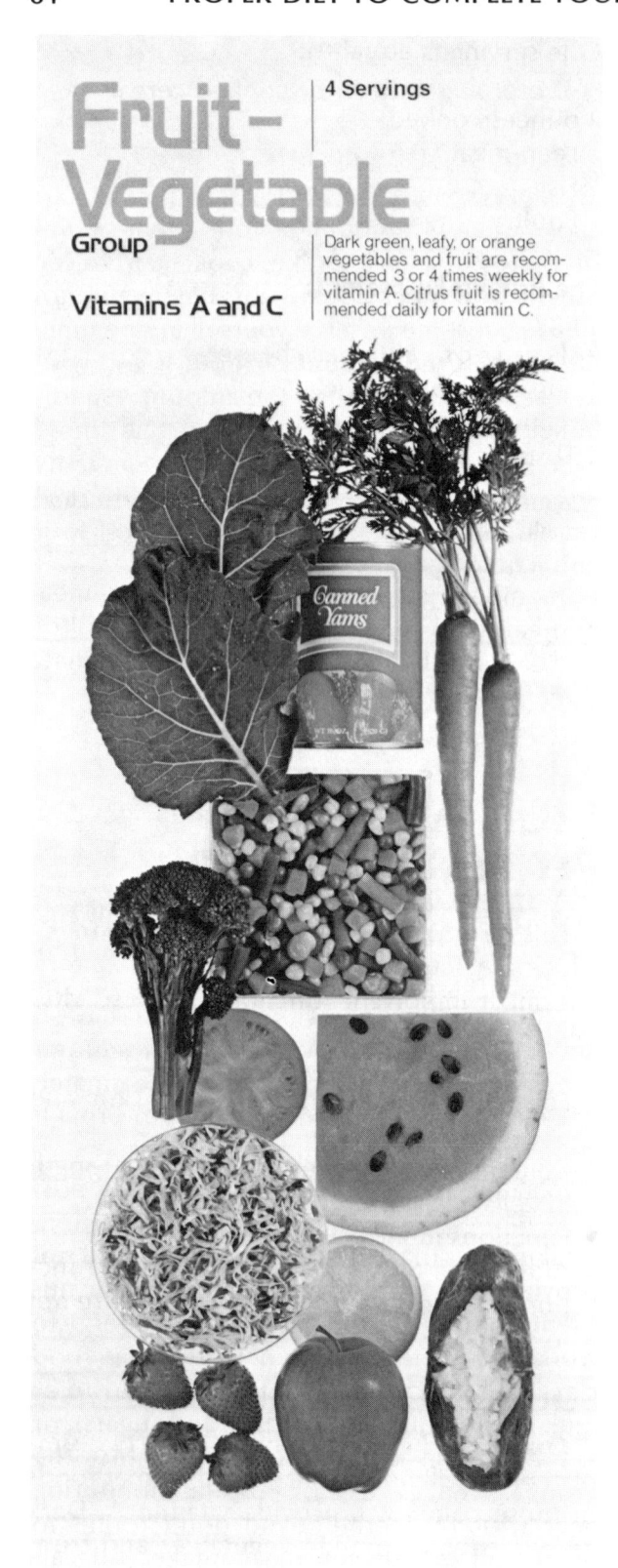

SOURCES OF VITAMIN C

Citrus fruits are recommended **daily** for supplying the needed catalyst, vitamin C. This vitamin is water soluble, which means that if too much is intaken, the extra is excreted out through the urine, etc. If you decide to take vitamin C supplement pills through massive doses, your body reacts by increasing the level it needs! If you suddenly stop taking vitamin C supplements then, your body reacts as if it were deficient! So supplementation is costly and unnecessary for well persons who eat right.

SERVINGS AND SOURCES OF THE FRUIT AND VEGETABLE GROUP

All persons need four servings per day. One serving is:

½ cup cooked
½ cup juice
1 cup raw
Medium size apple, banana, etc.[6]

Important sources of this group:

Vitamin A
Carrots
Sweet potatoes
Greens

Vitamin C
Broccoli
Orange
Grapefruit
Strawberries

GRAIN GROUP (Whole, Fortified, Enriched)

Although this group assists with the growth and maintenance of cells and with the elimination process (fiber provides bulk to your waste for easy removal), the major function is to provide energy. Your number one daily need is energy, to allow you to perform every single daily function, from sleeping to aerobic dancing.

Four servings per day is the minimum amount required by all groups. Remember if you do not:

- Use this carbohydrate food for the expenditure of energy

- Use it for growth and repairs or
- Eliminate it,

you **wear** it as **body fat** — future energy. It's like constantly carrying around extra gasoline for your car.

One serving is equal to:

1 slice bread
½ bun
1 cup cold cereal
½ cup spaghetti (!) or cooked cereal[7]
5 crackers
3 cups popped popcorn
 (minus salt and butter)

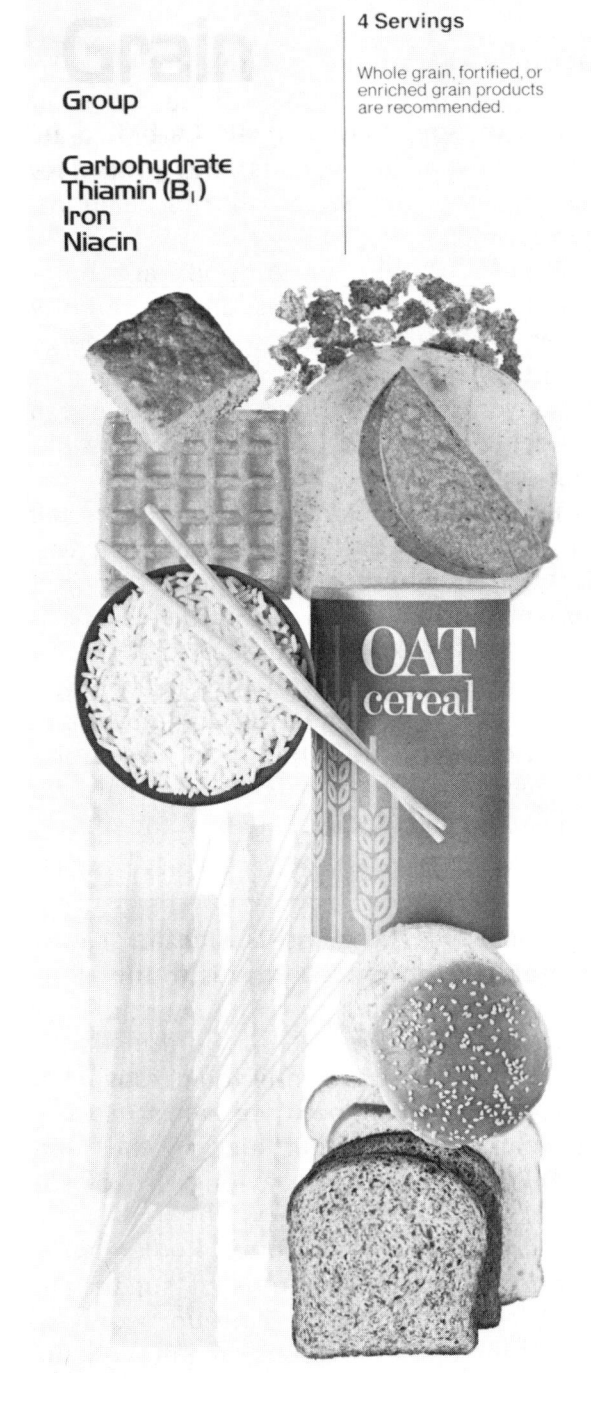

Grain Group

Carbohydrate
Thiamin (B₁)
Iron
Niacin

4 Servings

Whole grain, fortified, or enriched grain products are recommended.

A minimum amount of four servings was suggested as a daily intake. Look again to see **exactly how much** a serving is. It is, again, not all you consume or serve yourself at one time, but a **measured amount** of food. If you wish to lose fat weight, watch the amount of additional energy food that you intake. If, however, you are a quite active person — a varsity or endurance athlete — you will **want** to provide an abundance of this energy food **four hours before** your sport activity.

MONITORING YOUR INTAKE

If you intake an excess of food, good or junk, too much of anything will turn into fat tissue if it is not used or eliminated. If eating is your vice, and you don't like how all that extra energy "looks" on you, establish a monitoring program. Chart VII is a sample for you to follow. Write down when you have a serving of any group. When one daily column is filled, you have consumed approximately 1,200 calories, the basic minimum to provide for all the nutrients you need daily.

Intaking over this basic minimum will provide more energy to perform any exertion. Intaking less than this basic minimum will **not** provide you with all the needed daily nutrients to stay well and have enough energy to work and recreate. When you intake food classified as "Others" (usually referred to as junk food — high in salts, fats, and sugars), or extra servings of anything, list **below** the groups given, as "extra." Post the monitoring near your refrigerator, and don't forget to record **all** in-between-meal intake. All calories do count!

Remember — a "serving" is a measured amount — it's not all that you decide to eat at one sitting.

SPECIAL DIETARY GUIDELINES FOR AMERICANS

Food alone cannot make you healthy. But good eating habits based on **moderation and variety** can help keep you healthy and even improve your health. The following guidelines suggested for most Americans were developed by the U.S. Department of Agriculture, U.S. Department of Health and Human Services, and printed in more complete detail in the pamphlet "Nutrition and Your Health."[8] In brief, it is suggested that Americans need to pay more attention to the following:

①

Eat a variety of foods. No single food item supplies all the essential nutrients in the amounts you need. The greater the variety, the less likely you are to develop either a deficiency or an excess of any single nutrient.

②

Maintain ideal weight. If you are too fat, your chances of developing some chronic disorders are increased (i.e., high blood pressure, diabetes, heart attacks, strokes). To lose weight, increase physical activity, eat less fat and fatty foods, eat less sugar and sweets, and avoid too much alcohol.

③

Avoid too much fat, saturated fat, and cholesterol. If you have a high blood cholesterol level, you have a greater chance of having a heart attack. Populations like ours with diets high in saturated fats and cholesterol tend to have high blood cholesterol levels. There is controversy about what recommendations are appropriate for healthy Americans. But for the U.S. population as a whole, reduction in our current intake of total fat, saturated fat, and cholesterol is sensible.

To avoid too much fat, saturated fat, and cholesterol:

- Choose lean meat, fish, poultry, dry beans, and peas as your protein sources.
- Moderate your use of eggs and organ meats (such as liver).
- Limit your intake of butter, cream, hydrogenated margarines, shortenings and coconut oil, and foods made from such products.
- Trim excess fat off meats.
- Broil, bake, or boil rather than fry.
- Read labels carefully to determine both amount and types of fat contained in foods.

④

Eat foods with adequate starch and fiber. The major sources of energy in the average U.S. diet are carbohydrates and fats. Carbohydrates have an advantage over fats: they contain **less than half** the number of calories per ounce than fats.

Complex carbohydrate foods are better than simple carbohydrates. Simple carbohydrates (sugars) provide calories (for energy) but little else in the way of nutrients. Complex carbohydrates (beans, nuts, fruits, whole grain breads) contain many essential nutrients plus calories for energy.

Increasing your consumption of certain complex carbohydrates can also help increase dietary fiber, which tends to reduce the symptoms of chronic constipation, diverticulosis, and some types of "irritable bowel." There is also concern that diets low in fiber content might also increase the risk of developing cancer of the colon. Eating fruits, vegetables, and whole grain breads and cereals will achieve having adequate fiber in the diet.

⑤

Avoid too much sugar. The major hazard from eating too much sugar is tooth decay. The risk increases:

- With the more frequently you eat sugar and sweets, especially between meals
- If you eat foods that stick to the teeth (sticky candy, dates, daylong use of soft drinks)

Americans use 130 pounds of sugars and sweetners a year, each! (Line up twenty-six five-pound empty sugar bags to get the visual effect!)

To avoid excess sugar:

- Use less of all sugars (white, brown, raw, honey, and syrups)
- Select fresh fruit or fruit canned without heavy syrup
- Read food labels for sugar included — sucrose, glucose, maltose, dextrose, lactose, fructose, or syrup. If it's one of the first ingredients, there's a lot of sugar inside.

⑥

Avoid too much sodium. The major hazard of excessive sodium is how it affects your blood pressure. In populations where high sodium intake is common, high blood pressure is likewise common. In populations where low sodium intake occurs, high blood pressure is rare.

Sodium is in table salt (sodium chloride, both essential elements), processed foods, condiments, sauces (like soy sauce, steak sauce, garlic salt), pickled foods, cheese, salty snacks, sandwich meats, baking soda, baking powder, monosodium glutamate (MSG), soft drinks, and medications (like antacids). Read labels.

High blood pressure is a "forever" problem. Once you have it, you have it for the rest of your life and must **always** then monitor your sodium intake! Establish preventative measures early:

- Eliminate all salt use at the table
- Cook with no or very little salt
- Select foods that are low in sodium content.

⑦

If you drink alcohol, do so in moderation. Alcoholic beverages tend to be high in calories and low in other nutrients. Heavy drinkers may lose their appetites for foods that contain essential nutrients. Vitamin and mineral deficiencies occur commonly in heavy drinkers:

- Because of poor intake
- Because alcohol alters absorption and use of some essential nutrients.

It has been said that education leads to **moderation** in all areas of life. One or two drinks daily appear to cause no harm in adults. However, even moderate drinkers need to remember that alcohol is a high-calorie, low-nutrient food, and if you wish to achieve or maintain ideal weight, the intake must be monitored.

THE PSYCHOLOGY OF EATING

You eat to fulfill one of two purposes:

- Your hunger (physical need)
- Your appetite (mental need)

To establish a balance in your relationship with food, you must clearly understand **why** you eat **when you do.** To get in touch with this understanding is to truly "know thyself," and, for many people, to be able to make needed and wanted change in their overweight or obese bodies. For as it was discussed earlier in detail, nine out of ten persons whom we currently teach are overweight or obese and wish to lose weight. They feel that with aerobic dancing they will accomplish this. But the results of monitoring weight changes over an eight- to ten-week period show that only **very few dedicated** persons make any significant weight loss during an aerobic dance course.[9] By admission, they simply have not yet made the change in intake patterns both by volume of what is eaten, and also by selection of what is lower calorically. And, as previously mentioned, it is **easier to eat less food** to drop fat weight than it is to **exercise** it off, although a combination of both must be present to establish the proper kind of loss.

HUNGER VERSUS APPETITE

Physiologically, when you are hungry, your body will give you cues to "feed me," such as stomach pangs, perhaps a headache, maybe a weak feeling. It's time — time to take a break from the exertion in which you are engaged (work or play), relax, and **choose** wisely from the varieties that you haven't had yet today.

Appetite is mental hunger. You smell french fries cooking somewhere; you smell popcorn at the movies or ball game; you pass by a candy machine and "need" some energy; it's "noon" and you get an "attack" as you pass by a local fast-food restaurant; or you're watching TV and see your favorite food advertised. All of these **external cues** are **mental cues** — your **mind** is telling you that you are in need of food, rather than your **internal cues,** or **physical cues,** which show that true hunger is present and that nourishment is necessary.

Physical hunger can be satisfied by educating yourself toward your body's cues: "Boy, I'm hungry for a salad," or "A piece of meat for dinner must be part of my next meal!" You seem to crave a specific need. And when you have eaten enough, you have a "full feeling" and can continue on with your day.

Mental hunger or appetite can **never** be satisfied. Ponder that a moment. There is no bottom of the barrel — You eat, not listening to physical cues but to mental ones — and they never stop coming.

- "Here's a candy bar. It will make you (or me) feel better."
- "I need another glass of pop (coffee, etc. — caffeine), to settle my nerves."
- "I just exercised for a half hour, so I'm going to go "reward" myself with a big hot fudge sundae!"

Eating and drinking are used to relieve the **stress** that you are experiencing in life, today. Everyone does this at one time or another, but it is the vast majority of people who **regularly** eat to excess — three times a day plus constant snacking — that have the overweight and obese problem. And simply, if you don't want your reaction to stress to show on you like a flag waving help, you must select another outlet for life's daily situations of stress than eating and drinking! Hopefully, you will select a **positive** outlet for your stress like aerobic dance and relaxation, rather than an equally negative outlet to overeating (smoking, excessive drinking, wife-husband-child abuse, etc.).

ESTABLISHING CHANGE

Here are a few suggestions to make changes in your mental cueing (entitled behavior modification):

①

Establish (on paper) a list of your known food "vices" — those foods that you know are "bad" for you that you crave, right now.

②

When you see each of these foods, re-cue yourself by saying, "chocolate is manure;" "potato chips are broken glass;" "soda pop is bleach." Repeat and mentally "program" yourself to smell, taste, and **feel** about this product as you do, about the new cue — "It's bad for me. Why would I want to eat manure, broken glass, or bleach?" Your mind has capabilities beyond your comprehension! If you **really** want to change, you can. You must want to, badly enough, to try a new way.

③

Eat only when you are seated, relaxing, and enjoying this nourishment that you physiologically need. If it's at mealtime, eat only when you sit down with someone else, especially if you are a problem overeater. If it's a snack, determine by asking yourself:

- Am I hungry?
- Do I need this variety of food?
- How many calories is this equal to, in terms of how long will it take me to aerobically dance it off?

④

Think first, and then fill your plate one time with a measured (thought out) quantity that you need. Don't refill for seconds (that's mental cueing).

⑤

If food is left over, wrap it up and keep it for another meal or needed snack later. Don't eat to clean up someone's plate so it doesn't go to waste. It **goes** to waste — **your** waist!

⑥

When you eat or drink something, concentrate on what it tastes like, what it feels like, and what it's going to do for you. Take time to chew and savor. Don't just wolf it down!

⑦

When your hunger is satisfied, develop a new cue to stop eating:

- Place your napkin on your plate and fold your hands until you get up.
- Place your silver on your plate and "nurse" only a glass of water.
- Immediately chew a piece of sugarfree gum. Have it at the table, ready.
- Excuse yourself, get up, and go to a bathroom, and brush your teeth or wash your hands.

But, program an **ending cue,** always the same, to yourself — one that you **can** follow.

Thus, to make change, you must first educate yourself by **knowing yourself** and then re-cueing your desire for food:

- Make a vice list of cravings.
- Make a new cue for each "vice" food.
- Ask yourself: hungry/need/how long of exercise equal to burn it off?
- Quantity/volume — take just enough.
- Leftovers go to **WAIST.**
- Take time to enjoy each swallow and bite, and you'll have no guilt feelings.
- When you are done, do your new ending cue, everytime you eat.

"Oh God, give us
serenity to accept what
cannot be changed,
courage to change what
should be changed, and
wisdom to distinguish
the one from the other."

Reinhold Neibuhr

11

SPECIAL POPULATIONS, CONCERNS, AND MISCONCEPTIONS

As you go through life, you very likely, at one point or another, may find the need to reclassify yourself from a "regular population of aerobic dancers" category with virtually no limitations, to one who now possesses a special need, or concern. This chapter is dedicated to all of those fantastic individuals who are physically overcoming the **limitations** barrier because of less-than-an-optimum bodily condition. We've also included a section entitled "Special Concerns," covering the most frequent problems and injuries that occur in relation to this activity.

SIGHTLESS PERSONS

Sightless persons can aerobic dance, and Paulette, pictured here, is a living example. Sightless students mainstreamed into a conventional setting need several adaptations:

- A side wall to "trail" and hold on to at times while learning.
- Specific spacial boundaries that can be felt. Mats enclosing a wooden floor space worked well for us.
- Providing a cassette tape of the music with cues on it.
- The most significant aid is having an assistant in the class who is gifted in adapted movement. This individual can physically move each body part of the sightless individual through the range of motion being performed.
- Full-visioned persons rely heavily on visual cueing and correcting their body positions. Instruction to sightless persons must, therefore, be much slower, more specific, and much more detailed.
- It is quite difficult for sightless individuals to perform spacial moves (covering a large floor space, or up in the air). It **is** possible, however, to use a rope strung in mid-air about waist high in this person's area.
- This individual should concentrate on performing well about every third dance presented and work on perfecting one before another is begun. Later, during perform-

SPECIAL POPULATIONS, CONCERNS, AND MISCONCEPTIONS

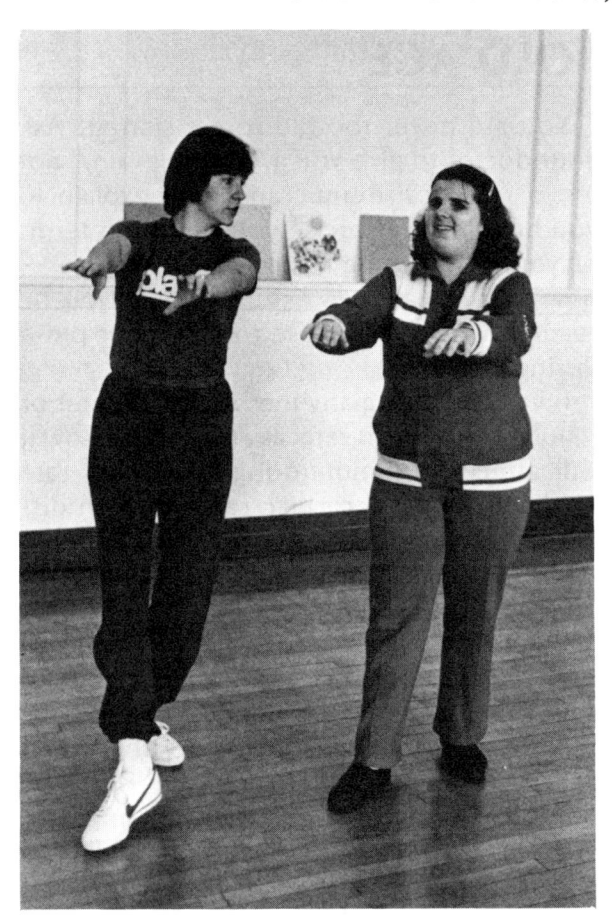

Full-visioned persons rely heavily on visual cueing and correcting their body positions. Instruction to sightless persons must, therefore, be much slower, more specific, and more detailed.

ance of those not learned, this individual should keep pace doing any aerobic movement — jogging or favorite steps.

AUDIBLY IMPAIRED

If you have a hearing disability, or are totally deaf, take a few pointers from Jane E. Herrmann, (now deceased) BGSU student of aerobic dance with whom we danced for four years.

①

Place yourself near the speakers and the instructor, and dance on his/her cueing side (the side to which cues are most often given when the group is not faced).

②

The instructor must **count out the beats** and **visually cue with finger counting,** at least initially. You must, therefore, make your instructor aware of your limitation, to assist your learning. Dances are totally learned by counting the beats, rather than the tune or words. Choreographers know that this is how all good dancers learn, anyway!

③

The instructor will assist learning if **transitional** head, finger, or arm cues are given for each sequence. Ask the instructor to do this for your benefit, if you are getting confused.

CARDIAC REHABILITATION PERSONS

Did you know that 80 percent of heart attack patients return to full and active lives?[1] But before starting an aerobic exercise program, **your first stop is your cardiologist's office!** Tell the cardiologist that you are interested is engaging in an aerobic dance program, and ask this doctor to define exactly your limitations. Ask and get answers to these questions:

- What are my limitations? List on paper.
- If taking medication, how does it work in terms of how my heart responds to it (goes slower, goes faster)?
- What heart rate monitoring (beats per minute) should I be reading to **improve** my cardiac condition?
- What are the **most** and **least** beats per minute that I should read in order to improve my condition aerobically? In other words, what is my "training zone?" **You must have a specific set of numbers (heart beats per minute) by which to exercise and dance!**
- A very small minority of cardiac patients are required to engage in **no** activity whatsoever. Am I a person who falls into this category?
- What outward body signs will I experience if I do too much exercise? List, so I can watch for their onset.

A physical fitness test (stress test) is the **best** way for cardiac rehabilitation individuals to start a program. You may be required to have an electrocardiogram taken at rest (no exercise), first. If this shows no outstanding irregularity, and it is assessed that you can safely participate in a physical fitness test (stress test), you would then be given a submaximal or maximal stress test. The exercise that you are asked to perform consists of walking three miles per hour on a moving treadmill, with increasing gradation of degrees every two minutes.

When and if your heart **starts** to show atypical electrical impulses, the treadmill is immediately stopped, and **below this is your maximum safe exercising heart rate.** You will not exercise at a higher heart rate until sufficient change has occurred and another treadmill test determines that you can do more work (exercise at a higher heart rate). So start your rehabilitation program the **right** way: begin with first a resting ECG and then a stress ECG to establish your limitations.

Cardiac rehabilitation exercise guidelines are:[2]

①

Work up gradually to the amount and type of exercise recommended by your cardiologist and physician.

②

STOP at the first sign of angina, fatigue, or shortness of breath.

③

Rest and take nitroglycerin if angina occurs. Report any concerns about this to your physician or health team.

④

Don't compete or push yourself. The desire to win may dull your senses to how you feel while exercising.

⑤

Do not exercise after drinking alcohol, after eating a heavy meal, or during emotional upsets.

"OLD AGE"

You are never too old to get started! Ask your doctor to give you a "fitness exam," not just a "physical exam," and then explain to you how much exercise you can do in terms of your monitoring your own heart rate — how many beats per minute should you be reading when you pause to take your pulse during activity?

If you are taking any medication to alter or regulate your heart rate, ask the doctor how it will affect your monitoring and pulse rate reading. (Refer to cardiac rehabilitation discussion for specific questions to ask.)

If you have specific diagnosed diseases that accompany the aging processes, like some forms of arthritis, ask how much is enough, how much is too much, and what kinds of pain (threshold) should be your guide. Basically, try to obtain specifics, rather than generalities.

Aerobic exercises are designed to increase the amount of oxygen used. Brain cells deprived of sufficient oxygen do not function efficiently, causing the powers of intellect and reason to fade.[3] Alertness and intellectual capabilities improve when the oxygen supply to the brain is increased.[4] Some experimenters feel that improved oxygen transport is the best deterrent to one of middle age's major killers — cerebral vascular disease.

To reduce the possibility of this dreaded occurrence, provide yourself with the physical stimulation necessary to promote more oxygen use by your body.

Here are a few guidelines for your physical fitness program:

- Medical exam a **must** before you begin.
- Totally individualize your program and gradually increase dosage. Perform slow and rhythmically initially.
- Warm up thoroughly.
- Controlled breathing (inhale and exhale properly) a must.
- **Interval training** is for you.
- No alcohol prior to exercising. It makes the heart work much too hard.
- Avoid arm-support exercises.
- Avoid isometrics.

Dancing Damsel is in Big Trouble

by Erma Bombeck

Confessions of an 8 a.m. Monday, Wednesday, Friday, Beginning Aerobic Dancer

"Oh, God, this was a mistake.

"I knew it. I'm the only person in this room who remembers Guy Lombardo and has backs of knees that look like a map of New England. Tens. They're all tens going on 15.

"Please, God, I have never asked you for a big one. If you remember the time I let my mother-in-law feed my husband hot soup a spoonful at a time when he had a cold and said nothing . . . let me have a spot in the back row. Now listen to me, feet, I'm going to tell you this just once. When that music starts I want you to move. I don't care what the rest of my body tells you . . . just move!

"Why me, God? Why do I always get next to the girl whose hair is long enough on top to pull back? Who doesn't wear underwear under her leotard? Who takes the chiffon scarf off her neck and ties it around her waist? Whose tights bag at the knees?

"The music is starting. Step, close, twirl, kick. Step, close, twirl, kick. Dummy! You just apologized to a wall for bumping into it. Wish I could take off these warm-up pants, but I don't know anyone in this room well enough to let them see my thighs.

"All this is my husband's fault. I used to dance until I married him. Now I've lost it. That's not the only excuse. I'm a mother. None of these girls in here has ever given birth. None of them knows what it is to dance when your entire body is arranged around your knees.

"How long is this record? What is she saying now? Don't forget to breathe. If I breathed any harder, I'd fog up the entire mirror.

"My leg! I have a cramp in my leg! Oh, that's cute. They're playing 'Staying Alive.' Is it my imagination or is everyone looking at me? What's the matter with these people? Don't they ever get tired? I got it. This is the road company of 'Chorus Line.'

"Wonder how old Scarf Waist is making out? It figures. She doesn't even sweat. Not one bead. Come to think of it I've never seen anyone over 5 feet 7 inches who sweats. How do they do that?

"It's over. I think I hurt myself. Wait a minute. There's someone who looks like she's passing out. Her hair is wild as an unmade bed, her arms are dragging on the floor and her pants are bagging.

"What kind of a creep would put a mirror in a room this small?"

From: *The Plain Dealer*, Cleveland, April 15, 1980

- Avoid overfatigue.
- Provide time to taper off and relax every session.

"BAD FEET"

You want to increase circulation to your feet and lower legs to make improvement in the area, so an exercise program to encourage this is for you! Purchase a shoe that provides plenty of absorption for stress to ankle and knee joints, and you will find that much of the misery will vanish! To understand specifics in purchasing proper shoes for this activity, take a moment now and read the section in Chapter 2 entitled "Buying Proper Shoes."

Ask your doctor or podiatrist specifically what you can do and what you cannot do, and then follow these special limitations as suggested. Other suggestions that may help:

①

During jogging type activities, run as follows: heel, outside of your foot, to toe. Jogging is a heel first activity, so don't run on your toes. (Many beginners make this very basic mistake!)

Figure 4.

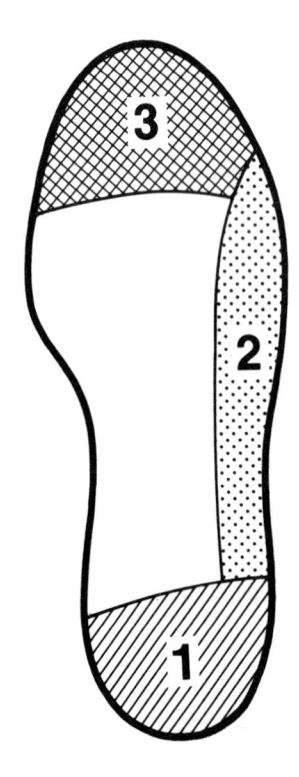

②

Dance on a **wood** floor. Tile or rubber-covered cement may add to foot/leg discomfort. If all you have available is a cement-based floor, buy a flat, thick, foam-backed kitchen carpet square mat (about six feet square), and dance only on this! Or even buy two or three, and stack them on top of one another. Bring them with you each time, if you're in a different facility than your home. You may feel apprehensive about taking this to an organized class, but if this makes you comfortable and able to participate — do it! Aerobic dance is an **individual** activity specific to the needs of each person, so do what makes you most comfortable.

PREGNANCY

Each woman should check first with her obstetrician/gynecologist and get this doctor's opinion on each individual case. Many doctors prescribe to this rule of exercise: You should be able to continue a program in which you have currently been engaged **before** pregnancy. If you have been involved in aerobic dancing (or jogging, swimming, cycling, etc.) you should be able to continue, but at a noncompetitive, lower intensity (pace of activity) level than previously done. This means less hopping, fewer lower leg and arm movements, and doing more stationary rather than spacial movements.

Dr. Michael Newton, M.D., professor of obstetrics and gynecology at Northwestern Medical School and director of gynecologic oncology at Prentice Women's Hospital and Maternity Center in Chicago, has enumerated the following guidelines to pregnant women:

①

If you have, prior to pregnancy, been engaged in an aerobic activity you wish to continue, are in good physical condition, and do not engage in competition, there is no reason why you should not continue your exercise program.

②

It is necessary to have an adequate diet, with

SPECIAL POPULATIONS, CONCERNS, AND MISCONCEPTIONS

emphasis on protein, along with some supplementary vitamins and minerals.

③

Physical ability decreases fairly rapidly even before the baby's increasing size makes great exertion impossible, so your intensity level will have to drop markably to coincide with this decreased ability.

④

Nonactive women are advised **against** taking up a new sport or activity during pregnancy, mainly because they would be using unaccustomed muscles and taking a greater chance of getting hurt because they will not have the necessary skills. However, if a woman is already athletically inclined and in good physical condition, there is no reason why she cannot take up a new sport in a moderate, noncompetitive fashion.

⑤

(Aerobic) swimming is a good exercise for the pregnant woman because so little pressure is exerted on the body, and it can be continued almost until the end of pregnancy.

⑥

Special problems that women experience during pregnancy are dizziness and the need to empty the bladder frequently. In later months, as the breasts become heavier, good bra support during exercise would become even more important. Increased lower back curvature occurs about the fifth month, with the increasing weight of the baby. Since your center of gravity is shifted forward, activities involving sudden movement might have to be reduced.

⑦

During the seventh month of pregnancy, the pelvic joints usually tend to become relaxed due to the rising levels of pregnancy hormones, especially progesterone, and some restrictions on activity would then become advisable.

⑧

Lactating women can continue exercise programs, beginning about three to four weeks after delivery. Women are urged to keep up an adequate fluid intake and a good diet.

⑨

Women who have Caesarean section can resume aerobic activities within four to six weeks of delivery, provided that their resumption of activity proceeds slowly.[5]

Many physicians are finding tremendous advantages in a good exercise program during pregnancy, since there are increased physiological and emotional demands on the body. A widely accepted aerobics program that is promoted by many physicians is walking. Make it aerobic by walking at the specific heart rate that is within your training zone, and you will have provided yourself with another option!

Several years ago, a study of Olympic women athletes showed that, overall, they had normal pregnancies and that no special risks or dangers were involved. Their improved muscle tone permitted them to complete the second, or expulsion, stage of labor more rapidly than other women. Recovery from childbirth was also better, partly because of the good dietary habits that these women had developed before pregnancy. (Some athletes have performed very well in the early months; however, Olympic-level competition is not practical during pregnancy.)[6]

Also, of late, some researchers have shown that aerobic activity (primarily joggers have been studied) may reduce the menstrual flow or show a marked absence in some females. If you are interested in childbearing, you may wish to consider this finding when beginning an aerobics program.

SPECIAL CONCERNS

The following concerns are those most frequently asked in an aerobic dance setting. Many of these areas deal with the care and prevention of athletic type injuries.

Your body functions in predictable ways, 99

percent of the time. If you understand cause, effect, and therefore **prevention** before the occurrence, you are going to find that exercising your body is not a drudgery of pain and injuries, but a joy — a release, an outlet, a diversion for the mental and emotional stress in your life. It feels **good** to be so "tuned in" to **your own** physiological needs that your risk of injury is low. This "tuning in" is not a mystical phenomenon but comes about by educating yourself about how the body works.

APPAREL AND INJURY

①

As previously detailed, proper shoes are your number one concern. When you jump or run, you place three to six times more force on your feet than when you are stationary. If you weigh 125 pounds, this means that you are placing 375 to 750 pounds of pressure on your feet with each jump or run. Your body can withstand the stress of exercise better if this extra pressure is "shock absorbed" by the shoe you wear, or the giving quality of the surface upon which you move. Select a shoe that totally supports your foot for aerobic dance. Criteria are listed in Chapter 2. Dance preferably on wood to all other surfaces.

And when its time to get a new pair of shoes, do it! The inside of the shoe deteriorates first, so gauge your buying by when the inside wears out, not by how the rubber on the sole, etc. wears.

②

You want to prevent friction, so wear cotton socks that absorb sweat and have no wrinkles.

③

"Leg warmers" (heavy, very bulky long socks that you will see performance dancers wear in-between performances) are for just that purpose. During the warmup phase of the aerobic dance hour, you may wish to wear these in cooler weather. However, while you are dancing, or in warm weather, do not wear them. You want to be able to sweat and allow your cooling mechanism to function properly. In order to sweat freely, you must allow the sweat to be on your skin, exposed to the air. Leg warmers will absorb sweat and not allow the cooling mechanism to function properly. When you superficially heat the skin for a duration of time, it retains the internal body heat and soon causes heat exhaustion or even heat stroke. You do not want to interfere with your body's cooling mechanism by the use of stylish fad apparel of any kind (the same principles apply to the use of sweatshirts and pants).

④

Tights or nylon hosiery are sometimes worn by women to aesthetically make their legs look better by hiding the fat or flaws located there. The only time that either (tights, nylons, etc.) should be worn is in **cold** weather to retain the body heat. Again, nylon materials (of which tights and nylon hosiery are made) retain body heat. In warm weather you must allow the legs to sweat freely by exposing the skin surface directly to **air.** Don't be embarrassed by how your legs look — at least you are **working on improvement** by aerobic dancing!

⑤

Finally, it is against all physiological principles to wear a towel around the neck during exercise. The major artery from the heart to the brain is located in the neck area and needs to be able to be cooled by exposure of the skin surface in that area to air.

BLISTERS

Blisters come in seconds and take days to heal. Even a small blister that goes uncared for will bother your aerobic workout. The best advice is to do everything you can to prevent them from forming.

Blisters are caused by friction — a surface of your shoe rubbing against the skin of your foot. Make sure that your shoes fit well — not too loose, not too tight. To assist in the prevention of blisters, one simple procedure is to lubricate the trouble spot with petroleum jelly before you put your shoes on for another aerobic dance hour. If you sweat a lot, powder your feet also. Improper fitting shoes are the culprit, so be sure that you do a few aerobic dance moves in your local shoe store to size up comfort **in motion** before you purchase the shoes.

If you get a *water* blister, care for it as follows:

①

Gently scrub the area with soap and water to thoroughly clean the area.

②

Gently swab with alcohol or a surgical preparation.

③

Make two incisions at the outer edges of the blister. Slowly press out the superficial fluid. Apply ointment or first-aid cream and bandage until healed completely.

If you get a *blood* blister, care for it as follows:

①

Ice the area.

②

Do **not** puncture. The chance of infection is great, since you immediately are in connection with your circulation system.

③

Place a "donut"-type compress around the blister until it is reabsorbed and completely healed.

CRAMPS (MUSCLE)

A cramp is a painful spasm of muscle. Cramping may occur during or following a vigorous exercise session and is the result of two different phenomena. Muscle cramping *during* an exercise session is primarily due to an electrolyte and fluid imbalance in your system.[7] Electrolytes are sodium, calcium, chloride, potassium, and magnesium. Cramping occurs primarily because you have not, with regularity, properly replaced your water intake as you condition and train.

If a great deal of sweating has occurred (eight or more pounds of water), replacement of those elements may be obtained by drinking, in solution (never in tablet form), a substance that replaces them. With moderate sweating and water loss, regular, daily water intake and proper diet will replace the needed fluids and electrolyte elements and do much to eliminate this type of cramping.

The most common cramps associated with exercise are those that occur in the twenty-four hours after exercise, expecially after having gone to bed and/or after a sudden movement. These cramps (postexercise) are not associated with electrolyte imbalance.[8] They are believed to be caused by muscle fiber swelling, causing then the agitation of (peripheral) nerves servicing the muscle tissue. If these cramps are frequent and severe, treatment is usually prescribed by taking .2 grams of quinine sulfate.

Immediate relief for either type of cramping is to static stretch in the exact opposite direction for a few moments.

SIDE STITCH

A side stitch is the sharp pain in the side and usually represents a spasm of the diaphragm, the lower portion of the breathing mechanism. It is believed that side stitches occur primarily because not enough oxygen is getting to the area. This is due to a decreased blood flow to the location and most frequently occurs in those who have recently had a meal or drunk large volumes of fluid.

To help alleviate this phenomenon, immediately inhale deeply and bend forward from the waist, making the stomach and intestines push up against the diaphragm, Then, "tune in" to your breathing and consciously control your exhale. Do this by forming your lips as if you were going to whistle, and exhale through your puckered lips about five to ten times. For some, this seems to help.

The more conditioned person rarely experiences this type of pain, so prevention lies in continuing your program with regularity, with special attention to strength activities for the abdominal area.

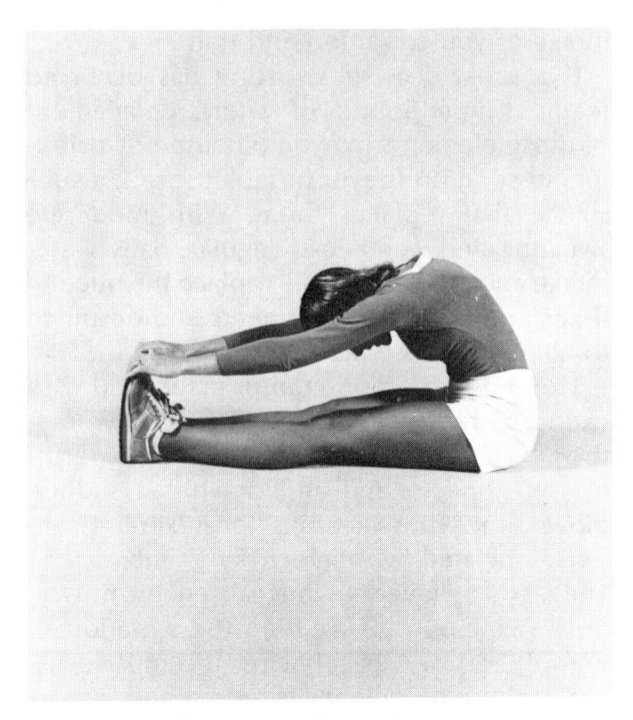

Exercise to alleviate a side stitch.

MUSCLE SORENESS

Two types of pain are associated with severe muscular exercise: (1) pain during and immediately after exercise, which may persist for several hours, and (2) a localized soreness that usually does not appear for twenty-four to forty-eight hours. The first is associated with the presence of metabolic wastes on pain receptors, the second with torn muscle fibers and/or connective tissue.[9] The immediate type need not be cause for great concern — it presents no lasting problems. The delayed type needs attention in the form of a more adequate warmup and cool-down stretching program, and the incorporation of concluding strength activities. Gradual, sensible muscle use during exercise is the best prevention.

MUSCLE, TENDON, AND JOINT INJURIES

①

For **muscle strains or sprains,** you I.C.E. = ICE, COMPRESS, AND ELEVATE. Injuries are iced (or cold whirlpools are administered) to inhibit swelling and promote healing by making the body internally (rather than at the surface) supply more blood to the affected deep problem area. The body forces more blood to come to the area when cold applications are applied by making the body work harder pumping away the old cells and pumping in fresh oxygen and nutrients to begin the repair process at the deep site rather than at the surface skin area. Ice applications are administered two times a day for about twenty minutes. When the affected area no longer is warm to the touch (using the back of your hand), but seems to be the same temperature as the rest of the leg, arm, etc., ice compresses can be stopped.

When heat is applied, it brings an increase of blood to the skin surface, but it doesn't make the body work hard at all — on its own — to pump in a fresh supply of oxygen and nutrients to the **deep** affected area. So stick with the less comfortable **ice** measure, and your repair process will quicken.

②

Achilles tendonitis is an inflammation of the thick tendon that connects the heel to the calf muscle. This injury is due to the use of shoes with inadequately thick heels, or which for some other reason do not provide a proper cushion for the foot.

To prevent Achilles tendonitis, perform adequate heel-cord stretching and **don't dance** with the pain. Aggravation of this problem can cause a serious and permanent condition.

FEMALE ONLY CONCERNS

①

To eliminate breast soreness due to the jogging-type movements performed, wear a **tight** bra (or jogging bra), and cover nipples with soft padding. Full-figured girls and women will find that a good supportive bra will do much to keep the breasts from early sagging, which is caused by the stretching of the connective tissue that provides the breast uplift. If you choose to wear a swimsuit for aerobic dance, again, remember to provide bra support.

SPECIAL POPULATIONS, CONCERNS, AND MISCONCEPTIONS

Figure 5.

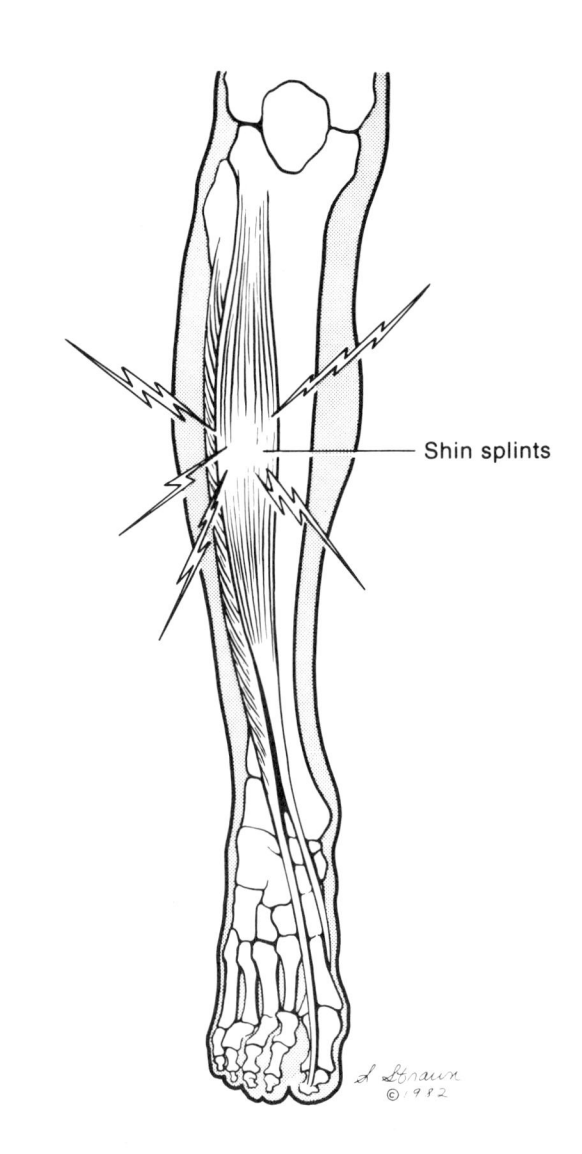

② Vigorous exercise will not make a woman's pelvic organs fall out or be damaged.[10]

③ Concerning that normal, monthly occurrence, the menstrual period — a program of physical exercise will probably help the occasional problem of menstrual cramps.[11] Circulation to the area is (greatly) increased with vigorous exercise, and therefore congestion is greatly eliminated, assisting in the alleviation of that uncomfortable feeling.

Also, exercises specifically designed for alleviating cramps are of **less** value than simply **practicing good habits of physical fitness and nutrition.**[12]

④ Menstrual abnormality (lighter flow, missed periods) is not unusual in endurance athletes. Some biochemical studies suggest that physical training affects the body's hormones, i.e., ovulation seems to decrease among runners.

SHIN SPLINTS

The most frequent injury experienced by new aerobic dancers is shin splints. The following information was provided by Jane Steinberg, an athletic trainer for intercollegiate sports at Bowling Green State University, Ohio.

"Shin splints is the term given to pain felt on the **front** and **inside** of the lower leg. Although a common affliction of runners, this malady can affect anyone who engages in physical activity which uses the legs. This includes aerobic dancers. Most cases of shin splints occur in the **beginning** of an exercise program because the lower leg muscles are weak.

Jumping and running activities cause the leg muscles in the back of the leg to develop and become stronger, while the leg muscles in front develop only slightly. This **muscle imbalance** can cause the disabling pain called "shin splints" if not treated correctly.

Preventative measures are the first step with any exercise regimen. Light, flexible shoes

— Shin splints

with good arch support are mandatory. Stretching before and after physical activity also helps the muscles absorb shock.

Performing three repetitions of straight-leg and bent-knee wall leans for twenty seconds may help alleviate the problem.

Of utmost importance in the caring for shin splints is **rest** and **immediately icing** the area of tenderness. The icing should be done for eight to ten continuous minutes by means of gently massaging the problem area. Later in the day, if time permits, a second gentle ice massage for the same duration of time should begin to give the desired relief. Continue this procedure for several days. You'll be amazed how quickly you "repair" within one week!

Straight-leg wall leans for relief of shin splints.

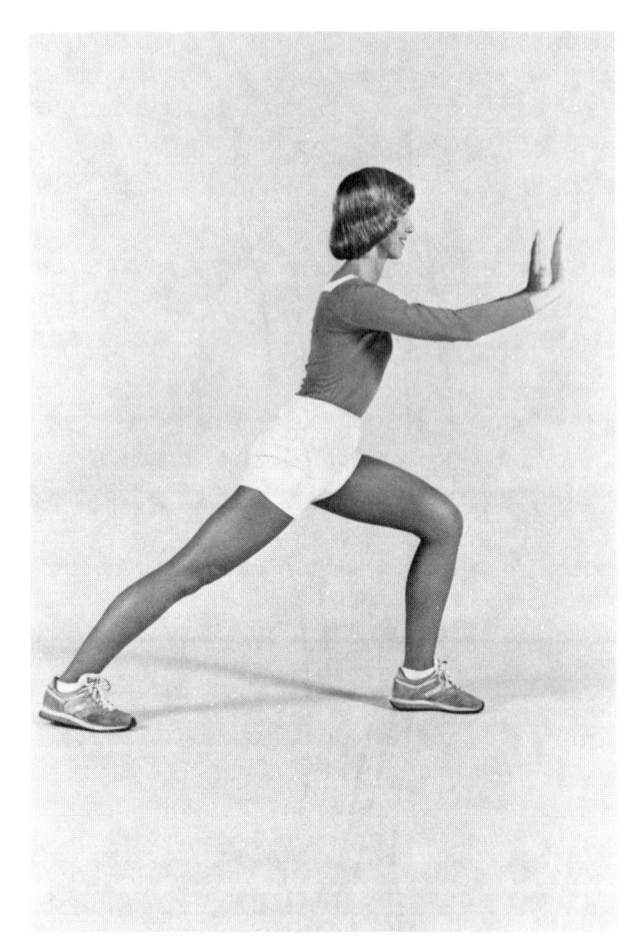

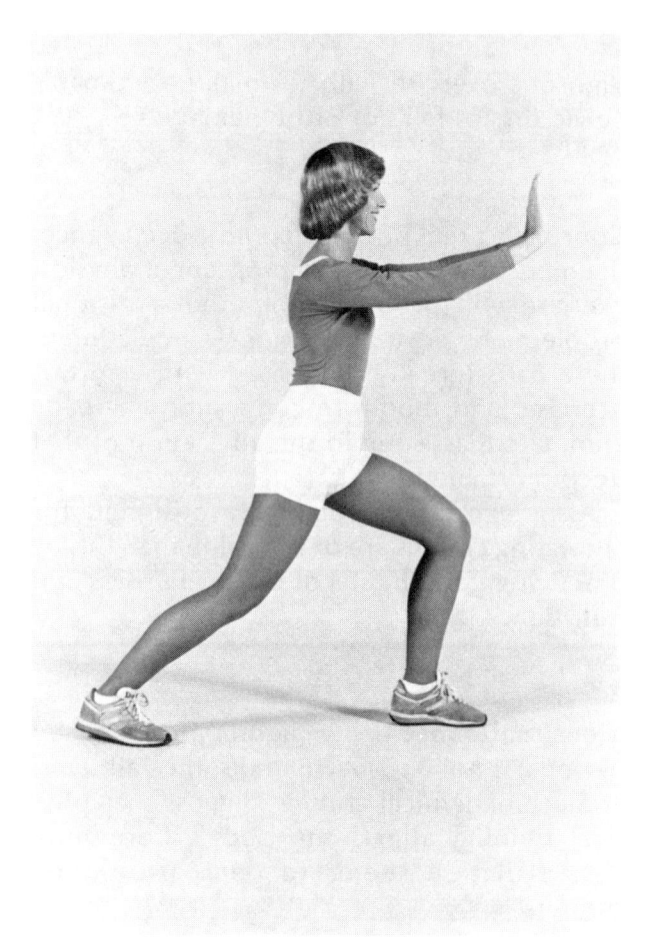

Bent-leg wall leans for relief of shin splints.

Also, you can minimize the discomfort felt by taking four to six aspirin a day. Toe raises on the edge of a step can help strengthen the posterior muscles which are heavily used in any running, jumping, or dancing activity. Walking on your heels with your toes in the air for thirty to sixty seconds is an easy way to build up strength in the front leg muscles. Pressing down on the heel of the fully extended leg while cycling also helps. Practice this stretch at traffic lights when you must wait.

If icing, rest, aspirin, strengthening and stretching do not create relief within ten days, see a physician to rule out the more serious conditions such as stress fractures, structural imbalances which might require orthotics, or anterior compartment syndrome."[13]

The "orthotics" mentioned above are angular inserts that fit inside athletic shoes to accommodate an individual's imbalanced feet, which can cause shin splints. The orthotic enables the individual's foot to land flat. You should have the advice of a physician or podiatrist before wearing orthotics.

WATER INTAKE

Being **able** to perform aerobic dance depends upon the replacement of your water losses. Water serves as the principle means of transporting heat (and substances) within the body. In warm environments (meaning within a room or a geographical location), it is the **only** means of dispersing body heat. This is accomplished by the evaporation of released perspiration on the surface of the skin. When the room air contacts the sweat, the skin surface is cooled, and the cooling is then internally conducted.

The production of body heat is greatly increased during physical exercise. **Unless water for perspiration is available, the body temperature increases beyond normal and there is overheating.** Thus, when fluid loss exceeds supply, dehydration follows, with an accompanying limited ability to exercise. When dehydration occurs, even modest physical activity causes the **heart rate and body temperature to increase.** When the water loss is approximately 5 percent of the total body water, evidence of heat exhaustion may become apparent, and when losses total 10 percent, the condition may soon lead to heat stroke, which is fatal unless cared for immediately (i.e., an ice bath submersion).

It is imperative that fluid intake be increased to maintain fluid balance as the work level and environmental temperature increase.[4]

Since there is no basis for restricting water intake during an aerobic dance hour and no evidence that humans can "adapt" or be "trained" to tolerate water intake that is lower than your daily losses, you should practice the habit of replacing water loss by continuous daily fluid intake.

Here are a few guidelines to facilitate water balance:

①

Drink plenty of liquids at least twenty minutes before the beginning of an aerobic hour. Frequent small intakes of fluid throughout the day is best.

②

For most sessions, if you have been providing plenty of water **prior** to the aerobic dance hour, you probably will not need to intake water **during** the hour (room temperature and humidity are the variables that usually determine this). However, if you get thirsty during an hour, **do not hesitate to drink water.** Your thirst mechanism is even a **late** sign that you need water, so don't ignore it!

③

After an aerobic hour, relax and sit with a tall glass of ice water or lemonade. This will provide immediate rehydration and is a pleasant way to conclude your hour "to yourself."

Deliberate dehydration (by loading on the clothes and promoting profuse sweating), of course, is not an acceptable method for weight control. This will cause a temporary loss of weight that is **rapidly regained by rehydration.** Loss of weight should only be body fat, **never** water or protein.

MISCONCEPTIONS ABOUT AEROBICS

Within any body of information, misconceptions arise from unresearched statements promoted by individuals **not qualified** to make the statements. So, **don't believe everything you read.** Select to believe authors whose credentials are impressive and who publish their findings in **professional** journals.

Whenever a successful (i.e., substantial interest and money profit is generated) new idea, program, or product comes on the market, it gains much positive and negative commentary. There will be people who agree with the principles of a product or program, and those who will have nothing complimentary to say, for whatever reason. There will also be a flood of get-rich-quick persons who market bits and pieces of factual knowledge interwoven with unresearched ideas, misconceptions, and plain false information!

Many of the myths about the harm that exercise supposedly causes and unscientific ideas concerning proper exercise and diet are being put to rest through better education.

This text has been written to assist you in understanding basic human physiology — how your body works and how to improve it in one very unique way. Our motivation is purely **educational** in nature. It will provide you with a firm base so that **you** can evaluate the various products and programs being highly promoted these days.

Our hope for the future is that you refer to the most qualified sources available to answer your questions on exercise and/or diet programs. People who are physiologists, medical doctors — especially cardiologists, athletic trainers, i.e., the **professionals who devote their entire working day** and lives to researching and understanding human physiology — are overwhelmingly more qualified to advise you on exercise and diet than a commercially orientated person. Glamorous personalities sell you on their knowledge with their winning smiles, their notoriety, and their price tag attached to their information. Don't be fooled. Follow the exercise and/or diet programs of the scientific professionals. Read only information from authors who dare risk the public challenges by **listing** their qualifications and their **credentials,** which show experience in the related field in question. You will then have provided yourself with the most up-to-date knowledge and a safe and fun way to good health. Good luck!

APPENDIX

EVALUATING YOUR PROGRAM

Improvement in your overall health after eight to ten weeks of aerobic dance can be personally evaluated by reviewing your progress in several areas: physical, mental, emotional, and social changes.

THE PHYSICAL ASPECT

①
What was your pre-program resting heart rate: _____; after just eight to ten weeks of aerobic dancing: _____.
Change: _____

②
What was your goal in terms of your weight: maintenance/gain/loss: _____

③
Did your eating habits improve; if so (not) how/why?

④
Rate your pre-program flexibility: very inflexible / inflexible / moderately flexible / quite flexible.
Rate your flexibility after eight to ten weeks: _____. What physical movement can you now do that you could not; or what goal did you achieve that you were working on? _____

⑤
Did you gain:
- Strength _____
- Coordination _____
- Self-confidence _____
- Better posture _____
- Agility (move quicker in all directions) _____

If so, where? _____

⑥
Do you have a better understanding of how your body works physiologically so that you can evaluate true or false claims, by products and programs, on exercise and diet?

MENTAL/EMOTIONAL

① Does aerobic dance provide an outlet for your stress? _____

② If you smoked, have you quit/cut down/stayed the same? _____

③ If you partake, does the consumption of alcohol or other drugs seem less necessary since aerobic dance has become a part of your weekly routine? _____

④ What specific psychological boost does this activity do for you, if any?

SOCIAL

① Do you prefer to aerobic dance alone, in a group, or both? _____

② If you were in a group situation, what specifically did you get from the group? _____

③ Did you make any new, lasting friendships? _____

NOTES

Chapter 1

1. Kenneth H. Cooper, Movie, "Run Dick, Run Jane," Brigham Young University, Provo, Utah, 1971.
2. Kenneth H. Cooper, *The Aerobics Way* (New York: M. Evans and Company, Inc., 1977), pp. 88-89.
3. Like the Student Recreation Center track, Bowling Green State University, Bowling Green, Ohio.
4. Like the Eppler South Complex track, Bowling Green State University, Bowling Green, Ohio.
5. Lenore R. Zohman, M.D., et al, *The Cardiologists' Guide to Fitness and Health Through Exercise* (New York: Simon and Schuster, 1979), p. 87.
6. Cooper, Movie, "Run Dick, Run Jane."
7. Ibid.
8. Cooper, *The Aerobics Way*, p. 10.
9. National Vital Statistics Division, National Center for Health Statistics, Rockville, Md., 1976.
10. Zohman, p. 72.

Chapter 2

1. The American College of Sports Medicine, Encyclopedia of Sport Sciences and Medicine (New York: The Macmillan Company, 1971), p. 216.
2. Lenore Zohman, M.D., et al, *The Cardiologists' Guide to Fitness and Health Through Exercise* (New York: Simon and Schuster, 1979), p. 81.
3. Unpublished research data collected on students of Aerobic Dance in the Bowling Green (Ohio) University and community area, 1980-1982.
4. Zohman, p. 87.
5. Michael Newton, M.D., Professor of Obstetrics and Gynecology at Northwestern Medical School and Director of Gynecologic Oncology at Prentice Women's Hospital and Maternity Center in Chicago, quoted viewpoints, June 1982.
6. Unpublished research data of Karen S. Mazzeo collected on students enrolled in Aerobic Dance courses.

Chapter 3

1. Broer, Marion R., *Efficiency of Human Movement*, 2nd ed. (Philadelphia: W. B. Saunders Co., 1966).
2. Metheny, Eleanor, Ph.D., *Body Dynamics* (New York: McGraw-Hill, Inc., 1952).
3. Wells, Katharyne F., Ph.D., *Kinesiology*, 5th ed. (Philadelphia: W. B. Saunders, 1971).

Chapter 4

1. Donald K. Mathews and Edward L. Fox, *The Physiological Basis for Physical Education and Athletics* (Philadelphia: W. B. Saunders Co., 1976), p. 103.
2. Carolyn O. Bowers, et al, *Judging and Coaching Women's Gymnastics* (Palo Alto, California: Mayfield Publishing Company, 1981), p. 335.
3. Bob Anderson, *Stretching* (Bolinas, California: Shelter Publications, 1980), pp. 9, 13.
4. Getchell, Bud, *Physical Fitness: A Way of Life* (New York: John Wiley & Sons, Inc., 1976).
5. Whaley, Russell, M.P.H., Ph.D., *Health* (Englewood Cliffs, N.J.: Prentice-Hall, 1982).

6. Allsen, Phillip J. et al, *Fitness for Life: An Individualized Approach,* 2nd ed. (Iowa: William C. Brown, Publishers, 1980).

7. Myers, Clayton R., *The Official YMCA Physical Fitness Handbook* (New York: Popular Library, 1975).

Chapter 6

1. Fall, Harold et al, *Essentials of Fitness* (Philadelphia: Saunders College, 1980).
2. Allsen, Phillip J. et al, *Fitness for Life: An Individualized Approach,* 2nd ed. (Iowa: William C. Brown, Co., 1980).

Chapter 7

1. *Collier's Encyclopedia 1981 Yearbook* (New York: Macmillan Educational Corporation, 1980), pp. 159, 333.
2. Unpublished research data collected on students of Aerobic Dance in the Bowling Green (Ohio) University and community area, 1980-1982.
3. Ibid., 1982.
4. Ibid.

Chapter 9

1. W. Sheldon, *Atlas of Men* (New York: Harper and Brothers, 1954), p. 120.
2. Handout of Dr. Richard Bowers, Director, Sportsphysiology Laboratory, Bowling Green State University, Bowling Green, Ohio, 1978.
3. Jack H. Wilmore, Ph.D., "Anthropometric Estimate of Body Composition," paper delivered in the Fitness Section of 1972 AAHPER Convention, Houston, Texas.
4. Donald K. Mathews and Edward L. Fox, *The Physiological Basis of Physical Education and Athletics* (Philadelphia: W. B. Saunders Company, 1976), p. 422.
5. Ibid., p. 423.
6. Wilmore.
7. John Derek, *Time Magazine,* November 2, 1981.
8. Unpublished research data of Karen S. Mazzeo, collected on students enrolled in Aerobic Dance, Spring 1982.
9. Unpublished research data of Karen S. Mazzeo, collected on students enrolled in Aerobic Dance courses, 1980-1982.
10. Jan Lewis, "Nutrition Notes. Dietary Guidelines 2," Bowling Green State University, Bowling Green, Ohio, 1981.
11. Richard Eppstein, Director, Better Business Bureau, Toldeo, Ohio, during a lecture to Karen S. Mazzeo's class, January 1980.
12. William Gottlieb, "A Lifetime of Fitness" (views of Thomas Cureton, Ph.D.), *Prevention,* December 1, 1980, p. 54.
13. Lewis, "Nutrition Notes 2," p. 6.
14. Kenneth Cooper, M.D., M.P.H., *The Aerobics Way* (New York: M. Evans and Company, Inc., 1977), p. 64.
15. Lewis, "Nutrition Notes 2," p. 4.
16. Ibid.
17. Ibid.

NOTES

Chapter 10

1. National Diary Council, "Guide to Wise Food Choices" B 170-1 (Rosemont, Ill: National Dairy Council, 1978), p. 4.

2. National Dairy Council, "Guide to Good Eating . . . A Recommended Daily Pattern" B 164-5 (Rosemont, Ill.: National Dairy Council, 1980), 4th Edition, 1977.

3. Ibid.

4. N.D.C. "Guide to Wise Food Choices," p. 1.

5. Ibid., p. 4.

6. Ibid.

7. Ibid.

8. U.S. Department of Agriculture, U.S. Department of Health and Human Services, Home and Garden Bulletin No. 232, "Nutrition and Your Health, Dietary Guidelines for Americans," February 1980.

9. Unpublished research data of Karen S. Mazzeo, collected on students of Aerobic Dance, 1980-1982.

Chapter 11

1. American Heart Association, "Heart Attack—What's Ahead?" Georgia Affiliate Inc., and Pritchett and Hull Assoc., Inc., 1980.

2. Ibid.

3. Paul Rosenfield, "Cooper's Cohorts Run Down Heart Disease," *Saturday Evening Post*, September, 1977, p. 20.

4. Ibid.

5. Michael Newton, M.D., Professor of Obstetrics and Gynecology at Northwestern Medical School and Director of Gynecologic Oncology at Prentice Women's Hospital and Maternity Center in Chicago, quoted viewpoints, June 1982.

6. Ibid.

7. The American College of Sports Medicine, *Encyclopedia of Sport Sciences and Medicine* (New York: The Macmillan Company, 1971), p. 215.

8. Ibid., p. 216.

9. Ibid.

10. Michael Newton, M.D., June 1982.

11. Ibid.

12. Ibid.

13. Interview with Jane Steinberg, Athletic Trainer of Intercollegiate Sports at Bowling Green State University, Bowling Green, Ohio, Spring 1982.

14. Committee on Nutritional Misinformation, Food and Nutrition Board, National Research Council, National Academy of Sciences, "Water Deprivation and Performance of Athletics," distributed by the Nutrition Education and Training Program, Bowling Green State University, 1981.

INDEX CARD OF INFORMATION: A PROFILE ON YOU

Name: _____

Section: _____

Index Card of Information: A Profile on You

In order to maintain a profile on students who enroll in a class, it is important to keep a few statistics so that change can be noted and statistics developed for future reference. Please fill in the following information, remove it carefully from the textbook, and give it to your instructor.

Name _____ Male / Female   Rank: F / So / J / S / Grad / Other

Address on Campus _____ Phone _____

Age _____ Height _____ Weight _____ Skinfold _____ Ideal Weight _____

Rate your Fitness Level: Superior / Excellent / Good / Fair / Poor / Very Poor — Pre
Superior / Excellent / Good / Fair / Poor / Very Poor — Post

Previous class or instruction in Aerobic Dance: _____

Sports in which you participate / Enjoy on a weekly basis: _____

Reason(s) for taking course: _____

Did anyone recommend this course or instructor? _____

Physical limitations _____

Activity that you would like for me to be sure to cover: _____

Heart Rate: Resting _____ Training Zone _____

Do you take any drug to alter your heart rate? _____

Do you desire to: (circle)   Gain lean weight / Lose fat weight / Stay same

Do you smoke? _____ If so, number per day? _____

Rate your alcohol consumption: Never / Daily / _____

Do you chew: Gum / Tobacco / Objects / Finger Nails

List interest in music, favorite song, favorite artist: _____

Other interests: _____

If age 35 or older, or have specific limitations: I have my Doctor's permission to participate _____

Doctor's name and phone: _____

I have read and understand the responsibilities for participants and the instructor.

_____   _____
Signature   Date

Name:_____

Section:_____

CHART I

Physical Fitness Appraisal Date:_____

Name: _____ Sex:_____ Age:_____

Appraisal was (circle): Before / During / After   Aerobic Dance Program

A. **12 minute** run/walk test on a **⅛ mile track:**

   Start Time: _____ Stop Time: _____

   Check Off Laps: 1 - 2 - 3 - 4 - 5 - 6 - 7 - 8 - 9 - 10 - 11 - 12 - 13 - 14 - 15 - 16 - 17 - 18

   Check Table I for Fitness Category.

B. **12 minute** run/walk test on a **.07 mile track:**

   Start Time: _____ Stop Time: _____

   Check Off Laps: 1 - 2 - 3 - 4 - 5 - 6 - 7 - 8 - 9 - 10 - 11 - 12 - 13 - 14 - 15 - 16 - 17 - 18 - 19 - 20 21 - 22 - 23 - 24 - 25 - 26 - 27 - 28 - 29 - 30

   Check Table II for Fitness Category.

C. Cooper **1.5 mile** run/walk test:

   Check Off Laps: (**14** for **⅛ mile** track; **22** for **.07 mile** track):

   1 - 2 - 3 - 4 - 5 - 6 - 7 - 8 - 9 - 10 - 11 - 12 - 13 - 14 - 15 - 16 - 17 - 18 - 19 - 20 - 21 - 22

D. Stop Time: _____

   − Start Time: _____   Just record here if
                                         using an open roadway.
     Time: _____

   Check Table III for Fitness Category.

Circle Fitness Category: Very Poor / Poor / Fair / Good / Excellent / Superior

Name: _____

Section: _____

CHART II
How to Figure Your Training Zone

Since two basic factors enter into figuring your estimated safe exercise zone, those must be established first:

1. Your current **age:** _____

2. How **active** is your **life-style?** _____% MHR. If you are:

   - Sedentary: use the figure **60-69%** of your maximum heart rate (but **only** for the first two or three weeks)
   - Moderately physically active: use **70-79%** of your maximum heart rate.
   - Physically active aerobically: **80-85%** of your maximum heart rate.

Now place your numbers in the formula that follows:

A. 220   - _____ = _____ Estimated Maximal Heart Rate (MHR)
    (index number)   your age

B. _____ - _____ = _____
    MHR   resting heart rate   heart rate reserve
                    (pp. 19-20)

C. _____ × _____ = resting H.R.   =
    heart rate reserve   lower end life-style activity range
                                (i.e., #2 above)

                                 _____ = resting H.R.   =
                                 higher end life-style activity range
                                 (i.e., #2 above)

RANGE OF   _____   This range is your **estimated safe exercise zone.** Keep your heart rate
YOUR   working in this range while you aerobically dance for the 20-30
TARGET   _____   minutes of each session of the dance routines.
ZONE

                         Re-figure as you "age," as you can reclassify your "life-style" of
                         activity, or as you have a marked decline in your resting heart rate.

For example: Chris is 20 years old, a moderately active person (70-79% range), with a resting heart rate of 62.

A. 220 - 20 = 200 MHR

B. 200 - 62 = 138 Heart Rate Reserve

C. 138 × .70 = 96 + 62 = 158   Training Zone Heart Rate
   138 × .79 = 109 + 62 = 171

If Chris keeps working (exercising) in the range of 158 to 171 heartbeats per minute, the heart would be **safely** working toward the training effect.

Name: _____

Section: _____

CHART III
Plot Your Resting Heart Rate

Establishing RsHR

WEEK I:

Day 1: _____
Day 2: _____
Day 3: _____
Day 4: _____
Day 5: _____

Sum Total: _____

÷ 5: _____ RsHR

Week	II		III		IV		V		VI		VII		VIII		IX		X	
Class	1	2	1	2	1	2	1	2	1	2	1	2	1	2	1	2	1	2

Bi-Weekly Resting Heart Rate ↓

120
115
110
105
100
95
90
85
80
75
70
65
60
55
50
45
40
35
30

NOTE: Take your resting heart rate at the first possibility in the A.M., before arising. Use first two fingers at thumb side of wrist, carotid artery in neck, temple area, or other pulse point.

Resting H.R. — Week I: _____ At Finish: _____ (−) Loss/(+) Gain: _____

Name: _____

Section: _____

CHART IV A
Monitoring and Charting During Aerobic Dance

Name: _____ Steady State: _____ Percentage _____

Starting Date: _____ Resting Pulse Rate _____

Date	Pre-Act. Pulse Rate	Activity Identified	Post-Act. Pulse Rate	Post-Cool-Down, Relaxation Pulse Rate

Name: _____

Section: _____

CHART IV B
Aerobic Dance Heart Rate Monitoring

Name: _____ Date: _____ Class: _____

Training Zone: _____ — _____ Initial Resting H.R. Average: _____

Directions: Check heart rate immediately after for 6 seconds. Add a zero and record as I reading. Keep walking. After one minute, check heart rate again for 15 seconds. Multiply by 4 and record, as "R" reading. First two weeks will include initial immediate readings which do not reflect the training zone (i.e., after flexibility).

WEEK 1		WEEK 2		WEEK 3	
CLASS 1	CLASS 2	CLASS 1	CLASS 2	CLASS 1	CLASS 2
Resting H.R.: 1__/2__/3__/4__/5__	_____	_____		Resting HR: _____	_____
Before Activity H.R. _____	_____	_____	_____	After Warmup I / R Jog/Rope ___/___	I / R ___/___
After Flexibility _____	_____	_____	_____	Aerobic Dances I: ___/___	___/___
After Warmup Dance _____	_____	_____	_____	II: ___/___	___/___
				III: ___/___	___/___
After Warmup Jog/Jump Rope I____ R____	I____ R____	I____ R____	I____ R____	IV: ___/___ V: ___/___ VI: ___/___	___/___ ___/___ ___/___
Comments:	Aerobic Dance Readings I / R I: ___/___ II: ___/___ III: ___/___	I / R ___/___ ___/___ ___/___	I / R ___/___ ___/___ ___/___	Comments:	Comments:
After Cool Down _____	Below 120? _____	Below 120? _____	Below 120? _____	Below 120? _____	Below 120? _____
Comments:					

	WEEK 4		WEEK 5		WEEK 6		WEEK 7	
	CLASS 1	CLASS 2	CLASS 1	CLASS 2	CLASS 1	CLASS 2	CLASS 1	CLASS 2
Resting HR:	___	___	___	___	___	___	___	___
After warmup Jog/Rope:	I / R ___/___	I / R ___/___	I / R ___/___	I / R ___/___	I / R ___/___	I / R ___/___	I / R ___/___	I / R ___/___
Aerobic Dances: I:	___/___	___/___	___/___	___/___	___/___	___/___	___/___	___/___
II:	___/___	___/___	___/___	___/___	___/___	___/___	___/___	___/___
III:	___/___	___/___	___/___	___/___	___/___	___/___	___/___	___/___
IV:	___/___	___/___	___/___	___/___	___/___	___/___	___/___	___/___
V:	___/___	___/___	___/___	___/___	___/___	___/___	___/___	___/___
VI:	___/___	___/___	___/___	___/___	___/___	___/___	___/___	___/___
VII:	___/___	___/___	___/___	___/___	___/___	___/___	___/___	___/___
VIII:	___/___	___/___	___/___	___/___	___/___	___/___	___/___	___/___
IX:	___/___	___/___	___/___	___/___	___/___	___/___	___/___	___/___
X:	___/___	___/___	___/___	___/___	___/___	___/___	___/___	___/___
	Below 120?	Below 120?	Below 120?	Below 120?	Below 120?	Below 120?	Below 120?	Below 120?
	After Cool Down ___	___	After Cool Down ___	___	After Cool Down ___	___	After Cool Down ___	___
	After Conscious Relaxation ___	___	After Conscious Relaxation ___	___	After Conscious Relaxation ___	___	After Conscious Relaxation ___	___
	Comments:	Comments:	Comments:	Comments:	Comments:	Comments:	Comments:	Comments:

	WEEK 8		WEEK 9		WEEK 10		
	CLASS 1	CLASS 2	CLASS 1	CLASS 2	CLASS 1	CLASS 2	List personal observations made on all heart rate monitoring:
Resting HR:	___	___	___	___	___	___	
After warmup Jog/Rope:	I / R ___/___	I / R ___/___	I / R ___/___	I / R ___/___	I / R ___/___	I / R ___/___	
Aerobic Dances: I:	___/___	___/___	___/___	___/___	___/___	___/___	
II:	___/___	___/___	___/___	___/___	___/___	___/___	
III:	___/___	___/___	___/___	___/___	___/___	___/___	
IV:	___/___	___/___	___/___	___/___	___/___	___/___	
V:	___/___	___/___	___/___	___/___	___/___	___/___	
VI:	___/___	___/___	___/___	___/___	___/___	___/___	
VII:	___/___	___/___	___/___	___/___	___/___	___/___	
VIII:	___/___	___/___	___/___	___/___	___/___	___/___	
IX:	___/___	___/___	___/___	___/___	___/___	___/___	
X:	___/___	___/___	___/___	___/___	___/___	___/___	
	Below 120?	Below 120?	Below 120?	Below 120?	Below 120?	Below 120?	
	After Cool Down ___	___	After Cool Down ___	___	After Cool Down ___	___	
	After Conscious Relaxation ___	___	After Conscious Relaxation ___	___	After Conscious Relaxation ___	___	
	Comments:	Comments:	Comments:	Comments:	Comments:	Comments:	

Name:_____

Section:_____

CHART V
Your Current Body Composition and Ideal Weight

Directions: Figure out your specific data and turn in to the instructor if requested for a course.

- Your current nude weight, in pounds: _____

- Your current skinfold measurement, in millimeters: _____

Wilmore's* formula for the anthropometric estimate of body composition:

Step 1 LBW (lean body weight):

Women:	**Men:**
20.20	22.62
+ _____ . _____ = (.635 × your weight in pounds)	+ _____ . _____ = (.793 × your weight in pounds)
_____ . _____ = a subtotal of above	_____ . _____ = a subtotal of above
− _____ . _____ = (.503 × your subscapular skinfold, in mm.)	− _____ . _____ = (.801 × your abdominal skinfold, in mm.)
_____ . _____ = LBW	_____ . _____ = LBW

Step 2 % FAT:

For Women and Men:

$$\frac{\text{Body Weight} - \text{LBW}}{\text{Body Weight}} \times 100 = \underline{\hspace{2in}} \text{ Current \% Fat}$$

*Wilmore, Jack, Ph.D. Director, Department of Physical Education, Exercise and Sport Sciences Laboratory, McKale Memorial Center, The University of Arizona, Tucson, Arizona 85721.

Categories:

Women		Men
30%	Obesity	20%
25%	Overweight	15%
22-20%	Ideal	12½-10%
Below 20%	Underfat	Below 10%

Thus, I am currently in which category? _____

Step 3 RELATIVE WEIGHTS FOR YOU:

Women:				Men:
$\dfrac{\text{LBW}}{.70}$	=	Your "Obesity" Weight	=	$\dfrac{\text{LBW}}{.80}$
$\dfrac{\text{LBW}}{.75}$	=	Your "Overweight" Weight	=	$\dfrac{\text{LBW}}{.85}$
$\dfrac{\text{LBW}}{.78}$	=	Your "High Ideal" Weight	=	$\dfrac{\text{LBW}}{.875}$
$\dfrac{\text{LBW}}{.80}$	=	Your "Low Ideal" Weight	=	$\dfrac{\text{LBW}}{.90}$
Below The Above Figure	=	Your "Underfat" Weight	=	Below The Above Figure

Thus, when you step on a scale and weigh the above weight(s) **at your current lean weight,** you can classify yourself into one of the four previously listed categories: obesity, overweight, high to low ideal weight range, or underfat range. The ideal percentage of fat to lean weight — called your "ideal weight" — is a **three-pound range,** not just one figure.

123

Name: _____

Section: _____

CHART VI
Plot Your Weight Maintenance, Loss, and/or Gain
(*Due this week of class.)

Weeks	I	II	III	IV	V	VI	VII	VIII	IX	X*
Pounds 15										
14										
13										
12										
11										
10										
9										
8										
7										
6										
5										
4										
3										
2										
1										
0										
1										
2										
3										
4										
5										
6										
7										
8										
9										
10										
11										
12										
13										
14										
15										
16										
17										
18										
19										
20										

Gain (lbs.)
Starting Wt.:
Loss (lbs.)

NOTE: Weigh yourself once a week, first possibility in AM, after elimination and before first meal.

Start of class weight: _____   End of class weight: _____   +/− Total: _____

NOTE: It is physiologically impossible to lose more than approximately 2 pounds of FAT per week.

Name:_____

Section:_____

CHART VII
My Daily Consumption

	TODAY	/	/	/	/	/	/
MILK							
1							
2							
MEAT							
1							
2							
FRUIT & VEG.							
1							
2							
3							
4							
GRAIN							
1							
2							
3							
4							
OTHER							
X-TRA							